WORLDWIDE WOUND HEALING - INNOVATION IN NATURAL AND CONVENTIONAL METHODS

Edited by **César João Vicente da Fonseca**

Worldwide Wound Healing - Innovation in Natural and Conventional Methods
http://dx.doi.org/10.5772/62668
Edited by César João Vicente da Fonseca

Contributors

César Fonseca, Tuhin Kanti Biswas, Chhaya Gadgoli, Philip Builders, Modupe Builders, Gilson Torres, Thalyta Cristina Mansano-Schlosser, Aline Maino Pergola-Marconato, Felismina Rosa Perreira Mendes, Eulalia Maria Chaves Maia, Sandra Maria Da Solidade Gomes Simões De Oliveira Torres, Dalva Cezar Da Silva, Rhayssa De Oliveira E Araújo, Abigail Gómez-Morales, Thomas Koob, Jeremy Lim, Mariana Carmen Chifiriuc, Mihaela Georgescu, Oana Marinas, Marcela Popa, Teodora Stan, Serban Vifor Bertesteanu, Veronica Lazar

Published by InTech

Janeza Trdine 9, 51000 Rijeka, Croatia

Publishing Process Manager Andrea Koric

Technical Editor SPi Global

Cover InTech Design team

First published December, 2016

Printed in Croatia

Additional hard copies can be obtained from orders@intechopen.com

Worldwide Wound Healing - Innovation in Natural and Conventional Methods, Edited by César João Vicente da Fonseca

p. cm.

Print ISBN 978-953-51-2805-2

Online ISBN 978-953-51-2806-9

For EU product safety concerns:
IN TECH d.o.o., Prolaz Marije Krucifikse Kozulić 3, 51000 Rijeka, Croatia,
info@intechopen.com or visit our website at intechopen.com.

Meet the editor

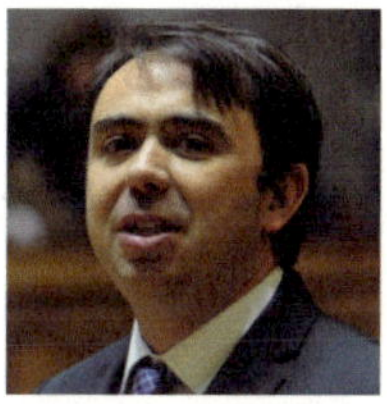

César João Vicente da Fonseca has received his master's degree in Health Communication at the Universidade Aberta and PhD degree in Nursing at the University of Lisbon. He is currently a professor in the Universidade de Évora. He develops the following thematic areas: evidence-based practice; clinical decision-making; clinical guidelines; care needs assessment, control, and eradication of pain; reflection of clinical practices; organizational management of social equipment intended for older people; and health indicators of long-term care organizations. He has played roles in coordination and control team of the research and development unit of nursing schools of Lisbon, being responsible for several epidemiological research programs in the field of public health. He is responsible for international publication of several papers and the achievement of several scientific meetings in the areas described above, with international impact. He is part of the Portuguese Health Systems Observatory. Some of the papers that have been published feature great international impact factor and international relevance. There are 150 citations of the article published in international terms.

Contents

Preface

I received the kind invitation from InTech—Open Science | Open Minds to write the preface of this book, so it was a pleasant surprise, a challenge, and a responsibility, because now this book will have its own life, with the aim of disseminating scientific knowledge throughout the world, according to scientific methodologies of several groups of researchers worldwide. The first reaction I had after I finished reading this book was joy to be in front of a remarkable work, based on scientific evidence that has practical use, with benefit for people with different needs of wound healing—a priority health care worldwide. This book is useful to practice care in chronic or acute wounds and for the welfare of the people and improving their quality of life.

Here, the purpose of the investigation is clearly demonstrated. All health care professionals recognize the importance of scientific development that has useful results to society. This book aims to prove the benefits of the symbiotic use of natural and conventional methodologies in wound healing. The caring of wounds is part of the health team action, where the major focus is clearly the persons/groups, their lifestyle, their quality of life, their aspirations, their potential, and their knowledge, which are the highlights of this book.

Worldwide Wound Healing - Innovation in Natural and Conventional Methods includes the identification and appointment of interventions in several chapters as in the "Efficacy of Traditional Methods in Wound Management in Africa," the "Journey through Ayurveda," the "Research in Phytoconstituents for Treatment of Wounds," the "Natural Compounds for Wound Healing," the "Nursing Interventions in Prevention and Healing of Leg Ulcers: Systematic Review of the Literature," the "Aspects Related to Venous Ulcer Healing and Its Influence on Quality of Life," and the "Placental Cells and Tissues: The Transformative Rise in Advanced Wound Care."

Thus, different chapters refer to the results of robust research studies, which are very important for showing the state of the art in the subject under study. The response to the desire of research results that have immediate application in care is now more clear. Rarely an immediate application is possible; the transformation/translation of new knowledge for each context is required. From the clarification of interventions to people with needs of healing complex wounds, the different studies help to understand the level of knowledge that was developed, the piloting of new intervention that already was constructed, and the assessment of the implications or this implementation in a specific context. We look forward to continued initiatives of this type, such as the new studies of the implementation of new interventions in wound healing with various global perspectives.

Enjoy your reading!

César João Vicente da Fonseca, PhD
University of Évora,
Évora, Portugal

Section 1

Scientific Evidence in Traditional Methodologies Wound Healing

Chapter 1

Wound Care: Traditional African Medicine Approach

Philip F. Builders and Modupe I. Builders

Additional information is available at the end of the chapter

http://dx.doi.org/10.5772/65521

Abstract

Wound care represents a major health burden in Africa. The types and causes of wounds in Africa are numerous; however, the interventions to these injuries are easily accessed in hospitals in the urban cities, while in most rural communities, the primary source of interventions is traditional medicine (TM). In recent times, there are incidences of preferences to the use of TM in the management of especially challenging wounds even when conventional interventions are available. In some African communities, there are incidences of quasi integration of conventional and traditional African medicine (TAM) in wound care. In the typical traditional African approach to wound care, diverse practices such as the use of herbal medicine, divination, and other physical interventions are common. There appears to be a favorable future for wound management using TAM with the increasing popularity due to various affirmative reasons other than poverty. The recognition, patronage, and uses of TAM for wound care as an alternative or complimentary to the conventional approach is expected to continue, hence, the need for the different regional governments in consonance with the WHO to promote the standardization, regulation, and other factors that will assure the safety and efficacy of the various practices and products of TAM.

Keywords: wounds, African traditional medicine, wound care, herbal medicine

1. Introduction

Wounds constitute among the major causes of visits to hospitals in Africa, accounting for about 30–42% of hospital attendance and 9% death every year [1, 2]. It is also among the most underreported health challenges in many parts of Africa, probably because of the poor access to hospitals among other reasons. In Africa as in other parts of the world, the causes of wounds are numerous varying markedly between age groups, environment, and occupation. Generally, the prevalent wounds in most parts of Africa are caused by assaults, road crashes, occupation-related injuries (in construction sites, farms, and domestic accidents in homes), animal bites, burns, surgery, and diseases (resulting in acute or chronic soft tissue damages). The primary source of interventions to wounds is the hospitals where health professionals are available to manage the different types of conditions as may be presented by the patients. An estimated 27–82% of the people in the different countries in Africa live in rural areas where hospitals and conventional healthcare services are either poor or nonexistent. Usually, the main option available to the majority of these rural communities is the indigenous traditional medicine [3]. The Africa traditional medicine has an intimate and long history of use and constitutes an important part of the culture and life of the people.

The various approaches to wound care in the different African cultures as shown by the knowledge, skills, and practices vary widely, and sometimes, with similarities that cross match in both far and near communities; nevertheless, the outcomes remain the same, which is, that the patients have quick healing and return to normal lifestyle [4]. In recent times, there has been an upsurge in incidences of preferences to the use of indigenous to traditional medicine for wound care even when conventional interventions are available. These arise due to certain experiences and prejudices that include perceived failure of the conventional therapy to meet the expectations of the patients especially as regards the management outcomes of such wound conditions as compound bone fractures, chronic ulcers, side effect of drugs, high cost of the conventional therapy, etc. [4, 5].

In the typical traditional African approach to wound care, diverse practices such as the use of herbal medicines, divination, and ritual performances are common [6]. The approach to the intervention often depends on the society, type, and severity of the wound. Generally, the use of herbal materials for wound management cuts across most cultures and wound types [7]. Though, much remain unknown about many of the traditional practices, techniques, and products used in wound care as regards scientific proofs that convincingly demonstrate the efficacy and safety of the practices, these traditional approaches will continue to play important roles in the healthcare needs of the people.

Sometimes, there is crude integration of the conventional and some traditional wound care practices. Some areas where integration is commonly used include in the treatment of bone fractures, burn wounds, and chronic ulcers due to certain diseases. In Nigeria, some traditional bonesetters enjoy high patronage. Some of the reasons adduced for this include claims of better treatment outcomes compared with the conventional approach, low cost, intimate interaction between patients and practitioners, among others. Many traditional medical practitioners (TMPs) integrate aspects of conventional healthcare practices such as use of antibiotics, anti-inflammatory drugs, and X-rays with their traditional methods in the management of certain wounds. Serious wounds such as burns, pressure, and chronic wound ulcers have continued to be the cause of morbidity and change in lifestyle of patients. Many of the difficulties have been tracked to the emergence of multiresistant strains of organisms to conventional antibiotics and the absence of effective conventional remedies. Recent scientific evidences and clinical trials conducted using certain herbal materials for wound treatment has shown good promise [8]. Some herbal materials including products containing *Hibiscus sabdariffa,* Aloe vera, and honey have been used extensively for wound care with excellent results [9–11]. The objective of this chapter is to have a comprehensive cache of information on the traditional approach to wound care in Africa. There appears to be a favorable future for wound management using the TAM approach. The recognition, patronage, and success of TAM in wound care as an alternative or complimentary to the conventional approach is expected to continue, hence, the need for the different indigenous governments in consonance with the WHO to safeguard the life of the people by standardizing and improving the regulation of the various practices and products used by the TMPs, design basic training (especially in areas of patient handling and hygiene), research and clinical trials to show proof of efficacy and safety of their practices, products, and techniques. This will ensure that only genuine practitioners are allowed to practice as well as ensure that only safe and effective techniques and products are used as a precursor to integrating this system into the mainstream healthcare system. In this chapter, the general concept of wound care, types, and efficacy of traditional interventions and indigenous African medicinal plants used for wound care are discussed.

2. Wounds

Wounds may be defined as a circumscribed damage that may be caused by physical, chemical, disease, or combinations of these factors often involving tissue or organ resulting in the disruption of the continuity of the epithelial lining of the skin or other tissues so that the integrity and/or protective functions of the tissue is compromised [12–14].

2.1. Causes of wounds

Physical factors capable of causing wounds are many. In ancient times, the primary physical factors that may generate wounds include battles, animal bites, farming, hunting, and culture-religious activities (such as circumcision, tribal marks, and body piercing), among others. In contemporary times, the common and prevalent physical factors causing wounds include assaults, road crashes, surgery, burns, freezing, corrosive chemicals (acids, basis, and so forth), radiations, animal bites, gunshots, occupational, and domestic accidents resulting in unspecified soft tissue damage due to cuts, abrasions, fractures, and so forth. In general, certain diseases including microbial, fungal, and viral infections as well as immunological defects have caused wounds. It is estimated that about 34% of all the diseases encountered worldwide are diseases with potential to cause wounds [15]. Common wound-causing diseases include diabetes, tumors, boils, athlete's foot, necrotizing ascitis, sporotrichosis, and chicken pox [16].

2.2. Types of wounds

Even in ancient times, people in Africa have differentiated their wounds based on their experiences from injuries incurred in their various day to day activities. The ancient Egyptians have differentiated their wounds simply into fresh and nonhealing wounds, which correspond closely to acute and chronic wounds, respectively, as classified in this contemporary times [17]. In contemporary times, however, the classification of wounds has become more complex so as to meet certain functional objectives.

Many wound classifications are based on such factors as etiology that relates to causes such as wounds due to mechanical injury (bites, cuts, abrasion, crush, muscle tear, incisions, and others), wounds due to chemicals (acid, basis, and other corrosive substances), radiations wounds, wounds from thermal factors (burns and freezing). Classification based on severeity related to physical presentation based on depth of the wound (superficial, partial thickness, full thickness, and deep wounds). Classification based on wound contamination (clean wound, clean-contaminated wound, contaminated wound, and heavily contaminated wound). There are other classifications that include surgical or traumatic; mild, severe, or lethal; simple or compound; acute or chronic [18].

In typical African communities, people sustain different types of wounds with varying severity in their daily life activities. Assuming the simple conventional classification of chronic and acute wounds, the common wounds encountered include incision wounds (e.g., circumcision), animal bites, cuts (sharp objects), abrasion, crush, muscle tears, diabetic ulcers, among others.

2.3. Circumcision wounds

Circumcision is a simple surgical procedure that results in an acute predetermined wound. In African communities, where circumcision is part of the culture there are always TMPs who are dedicated to this practice. They carry out the surgery and manage the wounds using traditional methods. In many parts of Africa, the traditional methods rely heavily on herbal materials and herbal products to prevent infection, ameliorate pains, and swelling, and accelerate wound healing [19]. Currently, conventional medical circumcision is popular in most urban African cities [20]. However, the traditional providers will continue to be an important approach to circumcision in especially rural area for various reasons [21].

3. Pains

Pain is an unpleasant sensation that is felt as a result of the brain's response to damage in the body [22]. It is an important feature of wounds. Pains due to wounds are usually localized, intense, and persistent, and may be exacerbated by physical and psychological factors. Most persistent wound pains may be related to conditions such as ischemia, hypoxia, venous insufficiency, vasculitis, or pressure. Conditions such as inflammation, hypersensitivities, and local infection can also result in persistent pains [23–25]. Pains due to physical factors are often related to movement, poor dressing techniques, and the use of inappropriate dressings, among others [26]. Psychological factors include factors such as anxiety, stress, fear, depression, and sleep disturbances [27–30]. Pains can greatly affect the quality of life of the patient as well as those taking care of the patient. Although it may not be feasible to completely eliminate the pain, however, an effective wound care system must make the pains tolerable [26, 31, 32].

There are two types of pains: nociceptive and neuropathic pain. Wound patients may experience both nociceptive and naturopathic pains. Nociceptive and neuropathic pains can either be acute or chronic; however, neuropathic pains are the major contributors to most chronic

http://dx.doi.org/10.5772/65521

pains. Nociceptive pains arise from damaged tissues and wounds such as compound fracture, burns, bruises, and inflammatory disorders are typically nociceptive.

Plant	Botanical part used	Common/ vernacular name	Type of wounds	Geographical/ country of origin
Acacia Senegal	Root	Gum Arabic	New wounds	Nigeria, South Africa
Aloe ferox	Bark	Bitter aloe	Burn wound	South Africa, Nigeria
Agathosma betulina	Leaves	Buchu	Open wound	South Africa
Aspalathus linearis	Root	Rooibos	All wounds	South Africa, Nigeria
Azardica indica	Seed	Dogonyaro	New wounds	Nigeria, West Africa
Bauhinia rufescens	Stem-bark	Danya	New and chronic wounds [33]	South Africa
Camellia sinensis	Leaves	Tea plant	New wound [33]	South Africa
Centella asiatica	Leaves	Gotu kola	New wound [34]	South Africa
Cyclopia genistoides	Leaves	Honey bush	New wound [34]	South Africa, Nigeria
Euphorbia hirta	Leaves	Buje	New and old wound [33]	West Africa, Nigeria
Hibiscus sabdariffa	Calyx	Zobo	Surgical wound [9]	Nigeria
Hypoxis hemerocallidea	Leaves	African potato	Wound heal	Mozambique
Merwillan atalensis	Bulb	Inguduza	Burn wound [8]	Swaziland, Lesotho
Moringa oleifera	Leaves	Miracle tree	New and old wounds [33]	Nigeria, West Africa
Musa sapientum	Leaves	Ayaba	New and old wounds [35]	Nigeria
Parkia biglobosa	Leaves	Iru	Chronic wounds [36]	Nigeria, Mali,
Pelargonium sidoides	Leaves	Umckaloabo	All wound	Senegal
Sclerocarrya birrea	Bark	Marula	New and old wound	Senegal
Siphonochilus aethiopicus	Rhizome	Wild ginger	New wounds [37]	Mozambique
Sutherlandia frutescens	Leaves	Petola	Wound heal [37]	Nigeria, Namibia, Malawi Botswana, Namibia

Table 1. Some indigenous African plants used for wound healing in TAM.

3.1. Nociceptive pains

Nociceptive pains arise from damaged tissues. Signals are picked up by sensory receptors in nerve endings of the damaged tissue. These nerves transmit the signals to the spinal cord and then to the brain, where the signals are interpreted as pain. The pains are typically well localized and constant. They are often described as aching or throbbing pain. Visceral (involve internal organs) and somatic (involve the body surface or musculoskeletal tissues) pains are nociceptive in origin. Wounds such as compound fracture, burns, bruises, and inflammatory disorders are typically nociceptive.

3.2. Neuropathic pains

Neuropathic pains are caused by either damage or dysfunction in the (peripheral and central) nervous system. The pain is frequently chronic and tends to respond poorly to treatment with opoids and nonsteriodal anti-inflammatory drugs. The pains are often described by patients as burning, tingling, shooting, stinging, piercing, stabbing, etc. [23, 24, 26].

3.3. TAM and wound pains

Herbal materials are the mainstay of the TAM approach to wound care. The holistic nature of TAM makes for a sensitive patient-centered care, whose goal is patient's comfort and accelerated wound healing. Most TMPs control wound pains by administering herbal materials or herbal products. Many of the herbal products used for wound treatment have combined immune-boosting, anti-anxiety, antibacterial, anti-inflammatory, and analgesic properties. The products may be administered orally or applied directly on the wounds [9] (**Table 1**).

4. Wound management with TAM

Some common paraphernalia used for wound care using the TAM approach includes divination, animal products, minerals, and herbal medicine. In TAM approach to wound care, the type of care and attention given to patients differ among the different people and cultures; however, factors such as perceived severity and cause of the wound are among the paramount considerations.

In especially chronic or serious wounds, TMPs employ their experience or use divination as a means of diagnosis to gain insight to the cause of the wound and also the probable remedy [38]. The healing agents may be applied directly on the wounds and/or taken orally or in a manner that the healer sees fit. The wounded patients are treated either in their homes or in traditional therapy clinics. In contemporary times, in the typical African rural community, wounds are managed by the TMPs with a salient area of specialization. For example, traditional midwives are experienced in taking deliveries and handling wounds arising from cuts and tears during childbirth, also TMPs specialized in circumcision, manage circumcision wounds. In most cases, the pedigree of the TMPs is well known by their communities and their client often repose a lot of trust in them.

5. Reason for the continuous sustenance of TAM

The status and practices of TAM in various parts of Africa vary widely due to differences in geographical, economic, and sociocultural orientation, among others. Indeed TAM generally occupies an important position in the healthcare needs of many Africans especially people in the rural communities. Sometimes the sociocultural and religious factors often have overwhelmingly influence on the system of healthcare. Many reasons have been tracked why many people in Africa continue to use TAM for their various healthcare needs. Some of the reasons include the following:

5.1. Personal preferences for TAM

TAM is an age-long system of healthcare that is deeply enshrined in the culture of the people. In time past, the people have relied on it as the primary healthcare system with much success. Despite modernization and the proliferation of the conventional healthcare system, some people still show personal preferences for TAM. This group of people will always prefer for their healthcare needs TAM whenever possible, and the choice exists irrespective of their financial, educational, and social status even though there are opportunities for prompt and easy accessibility to conventional healthcare services. The most popular aspect of TAM that is commonly used is the herbal medicine. Many people believe and use herbs, herbal materials, and herbal products as medicines for wound care and other ailments. The use of herbal medicine will continue to grow for many reasons: some people believe that herbal medicines are generally safe and carry no risk or side effect. This belief may be erroneous as many herbal medicines are comparatively more tolerable than orthodox drugs; however, they are not totally devoid of side effects, adverse reactions, and interactions with other products [39, 40].

5.2. Easy accessibility

In many African communities, there are inadequate conventional medical centers and healthcare practitioners as compared to easy and quick access to the TMPs. In many African communities, the TMPs generally outnumber the conventional health practitioners especially in the rural communities [41]. Many TMPs provide personalized, culturally appropriate, holistic, client-centered healthcare. In some cases, the autocracy observed in the attitudes of doctors and nurses may force clients to swing to the use of traditional methods. Also because of the high relative ratio of patients to conventional physicians, a lot of pressure is placed on medical personnel resulting in perceived or quasi-incompetence as many patients are often not satisfied with the attention given to them by health workers. The patients have insufficient time to interact and discuss their problems with their physicians and other health workers in matters regarding their health condition [42].

5.3. Low cost of treatment

The cost required to secure the services of TMPs in many rural African communities is often low when compared to that for the medical doctors. The TMPs are usually community members and are often within walking distance of their clients' and patients' homes, as against the long distances to be traversed to reach the conventional medical centers. The modalities of payment for services are often more flexible with TMPs, who may accept part payments or payment in kind (they may accepts chickens, goats, etc.) as against in conventional medical centers where the patients are often required pay before or immediately after treatment [43].

5.4. Efficacy of treatments

In recent times, there has been an increase in regulation and research activities into various aspects of indigenous traditional healthcare practices and products. The safety and efficacy of some products and practices have been scientifically evaluated and results collaborated with folk claims. The scientific proof of safety and efficacy has contributed to the increasing confidence and popularity of many herbal medicines and other products of TAM. There are also certain endemic diseases where patients have indicated preferences for TAM approach for the management instead of the conventional medicines [44].

5.5. As last resort

Some TAM practices and products are used as a last resort in the management of certain health challenges especially when the conventional approach has failed to yield the desired results. Some of such health challenges include chronic wounds, ulcers, and complex bone fractures. Indeed, sometimes the TAMs have proven to be better [45].

6. Factors affecting wound healing

Wound healing can be enhanced or impeded by several factors. The factors that can affect the healing of wounds can be grouped into systemic and local. The local factors include infections, slough and necrotic tissues, low oxygen tension, inadequate perfusion, foreign bodies, poor wound hygiene, and pressure, while the systemic factors include cardiovascular disorders, nephropathy, metabolic disorders (diabetes), high age, medication (e.g., steroidal anti-inflammatory drugs), poor nutrition, smoking, and immune suppression. Wounds under favorable healing factors will heal fast even with minimum intervention. In the holistic approach of TAM, some of the interventions are capable of addressing both the local and systemic factors at the same time [46].

7. Efficacy of TAM in wound management

Chronic wounds take a longer time to heal and may sometimes reoccur after healing due to overwhelming underlying unfavorable healing factors, hence, the need to identify such factors and treat them accordingly. Considering conventional healthcare approach to wound care, patients with chronic wounds often experience significant financial burden due to prolonged periods of treatment requiring dressings. There are claims of significant success when TAM was used as an alternative or complimentary to the conventional system of wound care. Some of the successes achieved by traditional bonesetters with various serious cases of compound fractures, diabetic ulcers, and burns in Nigeria highlight some of the achievement of TAM over the conventional [47]. Such feats have resulted in the popularity and trust in TAM interventions in the management of especially challenging wounds.

The concept of moist wound healing has been used to achieve effective accelerated wound healing with an added benefit of reducing scar. This approach to wound treatment has been recognized and practiced by many TMPs as shown by the use of various honey-based herbal products [48]. It is important to be continually conscious that TAM is a wide array of practices that differs in concept and efficacy along different cultural and geographical locations. The type of intervention and outcomes any TAM-based wound care system will achieve often varies depending on the effectiveness of the intervention [48].

Since ancient times, the importance of effective wound care and the benefits of maintaining wound-site moisture to ensure successful closure of the wound have long been known, as documented in the annals of the ancient Egyptians [49]. The target of an efficient TAM intervention to wounds is expected to have the following features: prevent and control of wound infections, accelerate healing, minimize pain, discomfort, odour, scaring, and protect surrounding tissues. This is achieved through the use of various traditional products that provide appropriate and effective physiological environment conducive for tissue repair and regeneration [50].

8. TAM approach to wound care

In the TAM approach to wound care especially as it pertains to severe and chronic wounds, certain practices and products such as divination, herbal medicine, and honey are commonly used in most parts of Africa.

8.1. Divination

In many parts of Africa, divination is widely practiced [51]. It is used as a means to understand the complexities of life and avoid catastrophe. It takes into consideration both the cause/source of the problems and remedies in relation to the physical as well as spiritual levels of existence to offer solutions to problems. In the management of perceived serious wounds such as severe burns and nonhealing wounds, some TMPs have employed divination as a means seeking information or direction for interventions or treatments from realms beyond the physical [52]. Thus, divination is a metaphysical practice used as a diagnostic tool in some traditional medicine practices.

8.2. Herbal medicines in wound care

Generally, herbal medicine is at the center of various interventions used in TAM approach to healthcare. Herbal medicines have been used as intervention in wounds by enhancing blood clotting, disinfect wounds, and accelerate tissue regeneration.

Herbal medicines include herbs, herbal materials, herbal preparations, and finished herbal products that contain as active ingredients, parts of plants, other plant materials, or combinations. Herbal materials include herbs and other substances such as juices, gums, and oils. Herbal medicines may contain plant materials other than the active ingredients and may also contain nonplant organic and inorganic substance as a component of the active ingredients [53]. The pharmacological activities of the herbs used in herbal medicines are due to the presence of bioactive chemical entities present as secondary metabolites. Some of these substances are capable of eliciting wound-healing activities among other pharmacological activities [9].

Africa has a wide botanical resource, and many have medicinal uses. Plants such as garlic, opium, castor oil, coriander, mint, and indigo were popular as medicines in ancient Africa. The African traditional herbal medicine is perhaps one of the oldest in human history. Many herbal recipes used in TAM contain herbal materials with alleged wound-healing properties. Empirical pharmacological evaluations has collaborated the folk claims of many of these herbs. The wound-healing activities of some herbs have been tracked to the anti-inflammatory, antibacterial, and skin-regenerative properties of their secondary metabolites. Some herbal products developed from traditional herbal recipes from various parts of Africa have shown to be effective in managing some challenging wounds such as pressure sores, burns, and leg ulcers that are often sources of intense pains and morbidity. These have proved to be extremely helpful in patients showing undesirable side effects or intolerability to certain conventional medicines. One probable important contributory reason accounting for the success of many herbal products used for wound care is their user-specific nature as most products are extemporaneously prepared to meet specific needs of patients. The extemporaneous products often do not contain any artificial additives or synthetic components such as preservatives, stabilizers, colours, or perfumes that may interfere with the activities of the active components.

8.3. Reason for the wound-healing potential of herbal medicines

Most of the herbal materials with wound-healing activities are known to contain biochemical substances such as vitamins, amino acids, fats, hydrocolloids, and some inorganic substances such as minerals salts.

The mechanism of the wound healing and other health benefits of the herbal materials have been tracked to their antioxidant properties [54]. The antioxidant properties of the herbs have been linked to their content of polyphenol and carotenoids. Antioxidants are classified into two major categories depending upon the nature of their chemical constituents namely carotenoids and polyphenols. Carotenoids are structurally related to vitamin A and constitute the various retinols like compounds. Polyphenols are antioxidant compounds that also include flavonoids. Flavonoids in addition to their antioxidant action also impart protection against ultra violet light and have metal chelating properties [55].

8.3.1. Polyphenols

Polyphenols are a large class of chemical compounds that are synthesized in many plants and are commonly stored in such botanical organs as fruits, seeds, leaves, and flowers of medicinal herbs, fruits, and vegetables. They are responsible for the colour, flavor, and healing qualities of many plants. They will inhibit the oxidation of other molecules. Polyphenols will terminate any chain reaction due to free radicals produced by oxidative processes. In many biological systems, such oxidative reactions often result in cell damage and other harmful processes such as abnormal platelet aggregation, which is a precursor to inflammatory responses. Flavonoids are the largest family of polyphenol compounds. Indeed, all flavonoids are polyphenols but not all polyphenols are flavonoids. The different classes of flavonoids include anthocyanins, flavanols, flavanones, flavonols, flavones, and isoflavones.

8.3.2. Health benefits of polyphenols

Polyphenols generally offer numerous health benefits [56]. As wound-healing agents, polyphenols will block the action of harmful enzymes that damage tissues due to UV radiations, wound ulcerations, and cell mutations by protecting tissue cells and body fluids from free radicals generated by oxidative processes. Some polyphenols have the ability to slow the growth of certain virulent viruses and microorganisms such as *Staphylococcus aureus* and *Escherichia coli*. Herbs containing polyphenols often elicit their wound-healing activities by such mechanisms as antibacterial, anti-inflammatory, and proregenerative activities. The antibacterial and anti-inflammatory properties of polyphenols will also prevent swelling and itching of the wounds by inhibiting the release and activities of allergic mediators such as histamine and serotonin [57, 58].

8.3.3 Sources of polyphenols

Many foodstuffs contain different types of flavonoids. Anthocyanins are common in many plants and are responsible for the characteristic purple and blue colours of many plants. Examples of foods rich in anthocyanins are blueberries, rossels, cherries, blackberries, plums, purple grapes, and pomegranate. Cocoa and cocoa products that are abundant in West Africa as well as green and black teas are rich in various catechins that belong to a group of flavanols. All citrus fruits and juices are also good sources of flavanones [59, 60].

8.4. Honey

Honey is the sweet, yellow- or amber-coloured, viscous fluid produced from nectar of flowers by bees and certain other insects such as honey ants and honey wasps. [36]. The taste and colour of honey may vary depending on what the bees are eating, geographical, and seasonal conditions. Honey contains high quantities of sugars and small amounts of amino acids, lipids, vitamins, and minerals. It also has good antimicrobial properties; hence, it can be stored without risk of spoilage [36, 61]. The wound-healing and other medicinal benefits of honey have been known for centuries in Africa and in many parts of the world. The medicinal use of honey by ancient Egyptians is well documented. Various empirical results have also shown the wound-healing potential of raw honey. The wound-healing activities of honey have been tracked to its antibacterial, immunomodulatory, and moisture-retention properties that enable it to disinfect, maintain a moist condition, and enhance tissue repair. The antimicrobial property of honey has been linked to the enzymatic production of hydrogen peroxide. The hydrogen peroxide disinfects and cleanses wounds. However, another kind of honey, called nonperoxide honey, displays significant antibacterial effects even when the hydrogen peroxide activity is blocked [62]. The antibacterial property of nonperoxide honey is related to low pH and high sugar content that imposes high osmolarity that hinder the growth of microbes [63, 64]. Surface skin wounds have been treated successfully with honey plasters with such benefits as reduction of pain and swelling.

8.5. Nutrition in wound care

Nutrition is among the critical factors that influence the outcome of wound care [64–66]. When injured, the body's metabolic process changes in attempts to repair itself. Such catabolic consequences often go unnoticed with good nutrition, and the wounds heal quickly. Poor and inappropriate diets can turn a normal superficial wound into a chronic wound since several processes including the body's immune capacity will be affected. Generally, nutrition has been shown to affect wound recovery time, tissue strength, and ability to resist infections. The consideration of proper nutrition in wound care has contributed significantly to enhance the healing of superficial wounds even with minimal direct attention. The practice of proper nutrition during wound care will make minor cuts to heal fast even without direct intervention as well as decrease the challenges, morbidity, and mortality often associated with serious and chronic wounds by reducing the impact, cost, and duration of management.

The nutrients that play important roles in the healing of wounds include protein, carbohydrate, fats and oils, certain vitamins, and trace metals. Protein is the nutrient that is responsible for the maintenance and repair of body tissues. Adequate protein levels in wound conditions will enhance collagen production and accelerate the wound-healing process. The amino acid L-arginine that is a block component of protein when taken as a supplement enhances wound healing [67, 68]. Proteins constitute an important aspect of the diet of most Africans and are derived from such sources as meat obtained from various domestic animals, *bush-meat*, and fish as well as various plant sources. Carbohydrates, fats, and oil are the classical sources of energy for the human body. These are obtained from various starchy, whole grain, and nutty foodstuffs. Energy is required during the anabolic processes in wound conditions for the synthesis of collagen. Higher carbohydrate and low fats heal wounds faster. However, the diet must be balanced as excess carbohydrates may also impede wound healing due to hyperglycemia [69]. The vitamins C, E, and A also play an exceptionally important role in wound healing. There roles are linked to the synthesis and cross-linking of collagen as well as the formation of new blood vessels (angiogenesis). Apart from these organic compounds, certain metals such as zinc, copper, and manganese occurring in trace quantities have also been linked to important roles in wound healing [9, 70–72]. Iron is also important and its role is linked to the perfusion of tissues with blood carrying enough oxygen to wound sites. Deficiency in these metals can impair wounds healing by impairing collagen production and strength of the wound [73].

The importance of these metals in the healing of wound could be the reason for the application of the ashes of the root, bark, and pods of certain plants on wounds in some folk medicine [2, 74]. Vitamins and trace metals are derived essentially from the various vegetables, fruits, and nuts that abound in most African communities. In debilitating wounds such as wound ulcers, diabetic wounds, extended burns, and amputation wounds, among others, diet control constitutes a vital aspect of the management regimen just as chemotherapy and dressing. Such wounds that affect especially the elderly, chronically ill, and accident victims constitute a large social, economic, and healthcare burden in many parts of rural and urban Africa.

Water is another component of nutrition and its functions includes hydration of the body to ensure efficient blood circulation that ensures that oxygen and nutrients are carried to every part of the body where the water is especially required for the optimal hydration to enhance wound tissue elasticity and strength.

9. Evaluation and authentication of claims of efficacy of wound care using TAM

Africa has a wide diversity of flora that is used for wound care. Various survey and review reports have established a bank of Ethnomedical information on the medicinal plants used for wound care in various African communities. Many of these reports focus on the ethnogeographical surveys of plant species and recipes used for wound care as well as reports on empirical research evaluations using appropriate models to prove the efficacy, mechanism of action, and safety of the herbs so as to corroborate the folkloric claims. Grierson and Afolayan, and De Wet et al . in their survey of medicinal plants used for traditional wound care in South African documented 38 species belonging to 26 families in Eastern Cape and 47 plant species from 35 families in Muputa land, respectively [75, 76]. Also, several surveys carried out in other parts of Africa including Cameroon, Egypt, Ethiopia, Ghana, Mali, and Nigeria have documented over 160 species from over 70 plant families that are used in traditional wound care [34, 35, 77–81]. These plants are prepared either as a mono-herbal or a poly-herbal some times in combinations with other substances plants. The herbs are prepared and used as decoction, infusions for drinking, or washing the wounds or are pulverized into powders to be applied directly on the open wounds, combined with other herbal materials such as palm oil, kernel oil, shear butter, etc., or made into poultices.

Due to the increasing attention in natural product research, a lot of work has been carried out to authenticate the various claims on the benefits of some of these plants for wound care. Empirical results have tracked the action of the wound-healing activities of some of the indigenous herbs to one or combination of the following pharmacological mechanisms: anti-inflammatory, antimicrobial, and cell-regeneration [82–85]. Many of these tests were carried out by simulating acute and chronic wounds using various simple animal models in rodents. The results have provided vital insights into the safety, efficacy, and mechanism of action of these herbs in wound care in relation to the type of herb and wound in a reproducible, controlled environment to corroborate or refute claims. The references to the authentications of claims of the wound-healing potential of some herbs commonly used in TAM are presented in **Table 2**.

Herb	Type of preparation	Type of test/mechanisms of action	References
Acalypha wilkesiana	Ethanol extract	*In vitro* antimicrobial, antioxidant assay, human fibloblast cell proliferation assay	[84]
Brideliaf erruginea	Ethanol extract	*In vitro* antimicrobial, antioxidant assay, human fibloblast cell proliferation assay	[84]
Dodonea viscosa	Ethanol extract	*In vitro* antimicrobial, antioxidant assay, human fibloblast cell proliferation assay	[86]
Ficus asperifolia	Aqueous	*In vitro* antioxidant assay, human fibloblast cell proliferation assay	[87]
Kigelia africana	Methanol	*In vitro* antimicrobial, antioxidant assay, human fibloblast cell proliferation assay	[83]
Lawsonia inermis	Methanol	*In vitro* antimicrobial, antioxidant assay, human fibloblast cell proliferation assay	[88]
Nauclea latifolia	Ethanol	*In vitro* antioxidant assay	[89]
Ocimum gratissimum	Ethanol	*In vitro* antimicrobial, antioxidant assay, human fibloblast cell proliferation assay	[84] [84]
Parkia biglobosa	Ethanol	*In vitro* antimicrobial, antioxidant assay, human fibloblast cell proliferation assay	[84]
Tridax procumbens	Ethanol	*In vitro* antimicrobial, antioxidant assay, human fibloblast cell proliferation assay	[84]
Urena lobata	Methanol	*In vitro* antimicrobial, antioxidant assay, human fibloblast cell proliferation assay	[90]
Vernonia amygdaline	Ethanol	*In vitro* antimicrobial, antioxidant assays	[84]
Ximenia americana	Methanol	*In vitro* antimicrobial, antioxidant assays	[91]
Zingiber officinale	Ethanol	*In vitro* antimicrobial, antioxidant assays	[92]

Table 2. References on the authentication of the wound-healing activities of some medicinal plants used in TAM.

10. Future of TAM in wound care

Wounds will continue to be an important health challenge in Africa as well as other parts of the world because of the contemporary complex lifestyles that predisposes people to physical injuries and diseases that cause wounds.

The orthodox health practice is the conventional intervention to wound care that has shown many successes; however; some treatment failures especially for chronic wounds have been experienced, which have been linked to factors such as high cost in treatment, severe pains, anxiety, and side effect of medications that have promoted poor compliance to treatment and resistance to antibiotics. The success in the management of challenging wounds using the TAM approach has been linked to the holistic patient care that centers on a flexible combination of potent herbal medicines, nutrition, good interpersonal interaction, and communication between the patient and the TMP and other desirable practices. Thus, the increasing popularity of the traditional approach to wound and general healthcare is fast shifting from the old reason of poverty to a conscious acceptance of the system even the eye of easy accessibility to conventional healthcare.

Increased regulation activities by the government of many African countries have resulted in increased standardization of various practices and products, proof of safety and efficacy, training of TMPs especially in hygiene, patient handling, and access to conventional health professional when necessary. The confidence reposed in TAM by users, the successful management of some challenges that the conventional approach has proved less successful, and the increasing resistance of many wound bacteria to conventional antibiotics have shown the potential of TAM as a health system for the future. However, there are still numerous important challenges about TAM that will need to be addressed before many useful practices and products of TAM can be used or integrated into mainstream health care system. Herbal medicines constitute a major component of TAM used in wound management, numerous herbal materials and products with promising wound-healing activities and folkloric claims are available; however, poor research and development and regulation activities of these products are not enough to assure safety and efficacy for its widespread use. In order to adequately harness these potentially useful products and probably integrate them into the mainstream healthcare system, various gaps will need to be filled and this includes adequate documentation on proof of efficacy and general safety including important adverse effects such as mutagenic properties and presence of heavy metal contamination, pharmacokinetic interactions with common conventional medicines, and robust clinical studies are necessary. There is also an important need for the promotion of research and development of simple, effective, and fast quality control techniques to standardize and to assure quality of the crude herbal materials and products, as well as formulating the products into simple, stable conventional pharmaceutical dosage forms. The availability of a large cache of potentially effective wound-healing herbs with evidence of antibacterial, anti-inflammatory, antipains, and antianxiety properties will serve as leads to the discovery of new compounds for the management of challenging conditions.

11. Conclusion

The population of the African continent is increasing rapidly, hence, the need to strengthen its healthcare system. One important way to do this is to facilitate standardization and strict regulation of indigenous practices and products that are potentially effective and safe. Indeed, the popularity of TAM in wound care as in other healthcare needs will continue to grow for various reasons other than poverty. Thus, there is an urgent need for the various African governments and WHO to encourage research and development of safe and effective products, introduce simple and effective quality control techniques that can be used to assure the quality of the various practices and products used in traditional medicine for wounds as well as for general healthcare so as to safeguard the health and lives of the people as a precursor to integrating the system into the mainstream healthcare.

Author details

Philip F. Builders[1*] and Modupe I. Builders[2]

*Address all correspondence to: philsonsky@yahoo.com

1 Department of Pharmaceutical Technology and Raw Materials Development, National Institute for Pharmaceutical Research and Development, Abuja, Nigeria

2 Department of Pharmacology and Therapeutics, College of Health Sciences, Bingham University, Jos, Nigeria

References

[1] Norman R, Matzopoulos R, Groenewald P, Bradshaw D. The high burden of injuries in South Africa. Bull World Health Org. 2006. http://www.who.int/bulletin/volumes/85/9/06-037184/en/.

[2] Adigun IA, Rahman GA, Yusuf IF, Ofoegbu CKF. The point prevalence and cost of wound management in a Nigerian teaching hospital. Nig Med J. 2010; 51(1): 23–25.

[3] World Health Organization. Fact sheet N134 Revised. May 2003. http://www.who.int/mediacentre/factsheets/2003/fs134/en/.

[4] Builders PF, Alalor CC, Avbunudiogba JA, Justice IE. Survey on the pharmaceutical quality of herbal medicines sold in Nigeria. J Appl Pharm Sci. 2015; 5(6): 097–103.

[5] WHO/EDM/TRM/2002.1. pp.1–74

[6] Mhame PP, Busia K, Kasilo OMJ. Clinical practices of African traditional medicine. African Health Monitor. 2010; 13. Accessed 20 April 2016. https://www.aho.afro.who.int/en/ahm/issue/13/reports/clinical-practices-african-traditional-medicine.

[7] Davis T. Traditional African healing. Accessed 20 April 2016. http://www.africanholocaust.net/news_ah/traditionalhealing.html.

[8] Dorai AA. Wound care with traditional, complementary and alternative medicine. Indian J Plast Surg. 2012; 45(2): 418–424. DOI: 10.4103/0970-0358.101331

[9] Builders PF, Kabele-toge B, Builders M, Chindo BA, Anwunobi PA, Isimi YC. Wound healing potential of formulated extract from *Hibiscus sabdariffa* calyx. Indian J Pharm Sci. 2013; 75(1): 45–52.

[10] Fawzi MM. Traditional medicines in Africa: an appraisal of ten potent African medicinal plants. Evid Comp Alternat Med. 2013; 2013: 1–14.

[11] Adib-Hashemi F, Farahmand F, Hesari SF, Rezakhaniha B, Fallah E, Fayyaz AF, Dadpay M. Anti-inflammatory and protective investigations on the effects of Theranekron® "an alcoholic extract of the Tarantula cubensis" on wound healing of peritoneal in the rat: an *in vivo* comparative study. Diagn Pathol. 2015; 10: 19. DOI: 10.1186/s13000-015-0252-x

[12] Pierce GF, Mustoe TA. Pharmacologic enhancement of wound healing. Annu Rev Med. 1995; 46: 467–481.

[13] Kumarasamyraja D, Jeganathan NS, Manavalan R. Review on medicinal plants with potential wound healing activity. Int J Pharm Sci. 2012; 4: 105–111.

[14] Mallefet P, Dweck CA. Mechanisms involved in wound healing. Biomed Sci. 2008; 10 (19): 609–615. file:///C:/Users/Dr.%20Builders/Downloads/2008-july-wound.pdf.

[15] Abbasi AM, Khan MA, Ahmad M, Zafar M, Jahan S, Sultana S. Ethnopharmacological application of medicinal plants to cure skin diseases and in folk cosmetics among the tribal communities of north-west Frontier province, Pakistan. J Ethnopharmacol. 2010; 128: 322–335.

[16] Solanki R, Nagori BP. A review on microorganisms causing wound infections on skin. Asian J Pharm Tech. 2013; 3 (3): 119–122.

[17] Margaret A, Lazarus GS Cowan DA, Aronson-Cook B, Kohli AR, Mamelak AJ. Treating the chronic wound: a practical approach to the care of nonhealing wounds and wound care dressings. J Am Acad Dermatol. 2008; 58 (2): 185–206. DOI: 10.1016/j.jaad.2007.08.048.

[18] Whitney J. Overview: acute and chronic wounds. Nurs Clin N Am. 2005; 40 (2): 191–205.

[19] Wilcken A, Keil T, Dick B. Traditional male circumcision in eastern and southern Africa: a systematic review of prevalence and complications. Bull World Health Org. 2010; 88: 907–914. DOI: 10.2471/BLT.09.072975

[20] Magoha GAO. Circumcision in various Nigerian and Kenyan hospitals. East Afr Med J. 1999; 76: 583–586. pmid:10734511.

[21] Berdeu D, Sauze L, Ha-Vinh P, Blum-Boisgard C. Cost-effectiveness analysis of treatments for phimosis: a comparison of surgical and medicinal approaches and their economic effect. BJU Int. 2001; 87 (3): 239–244.

[22] Builders MI, Okonta JM, Aguwa CN. Prescription patterns of analgesics in a community hospital in Nsukka. J Pharm Sci Res. 2011; 3: 1593–1598.

[23] World union of wound healing societies. Principles of best practice: minimizing pain and wound dressing-related procedures. A consensus document. London: MEP. 2004.

[24] Mudge E, Orsted H. Wound infection and pain management made easy. Wounds Int. 2010; 1: 3. tinyurl.com/WI-wound- Pain

[25] European wound management association, Position document. Management of wound infection. London: MEP.EWMA. 2006.

[26] Vuolo JC. Wound-related pain: key sources and triggers. Br J Nurs. 2009; 18: 15, S20–S25.

[27] Mudge E, Spanou C, Price PA. Focus group study into patients' perception of chronic wound pain. Wounds UK. 2008; 4 (2): 21–28.

[28] Soon K, Acton C. Pain-induced stress: a barrier to wound healing. Wounds UK. 2006; 2 (4): 92–101.

[29] Cutting KF, White RJ, Mahoney P, Harding KG. Clinical identification of wound infection: a Delphi approach. In: *EWMA* position document—identifying criteria for wound infection. London: MEP Ltd. 2005. 6–9.

[30] Doyle D, Hanks GWC, MacDonald N. Ed. Oxford Textbook of Palliative Medicine. Oxford: Oxford University Press. 1999. 3.

[31] McMullen M. The relationship between pain and leg ulcers: a critical review. Br J Nurs. 2004; 13 (19): S30–S64.

[32] European Wound Management Association. Position document: understanding wound pain and trauma: an international perspective. London: MEP. 2002.

[33] Rawat S, Singh R, Thakur P, Kaur S, Semwal A. Wound healing agents from medicinal plants: a review. Asian Pac J Trop Biomed. 2012; S1910–S1917.

[34] De-Wet H, Nciki S, van Vuuren SF. Medicinal plants used for the treatment of various skin disorders by a rural community in northern Maputaland, South Africa. J Ethnobiol Ethnomed. 2013; 9 (51). http://www.ethnobiomed.com/content/9/1/51.

[35] Grierson DS, Afolayan AJ. An ethnobotanical study of plants used for the treatment of wounds in the Eastern Cape. S Afr J Ethnopharmacol. 1999; 67: 327–332.

[36] Builders MI. *Parkia biglobosa* (African locust bean tree). World J Pharm Res. 2014; 3: 1672–1682.

[37] Street RA, Prinsloo G. Commercially important medicinal plants of South Africa: a review. J Chem. 2013; 1–16.

[38] Smith HS, Opioids and neuropathic pain. Pain Phys. 2012; 15: ES93–ES110. ISSN 2150-1149.

[39] McNicol ED, Midbari A, Eisenberg E. Opioids for neuropathic pain. Cochrane Database Sys Rev. 2013; 29 (8). DOI: 10.1002/14651858.CD006146.pub2.

[40] Omonzejele PF. African concepts of health, disease, and treatment: an ethical enquiry. Explore (NY). 2008; 4 (2): 120–126

[41] Shaw D, Graeme L, Pierre D, Elizabeth W, Kelvin C. Pharmacovigilance of herbal medicine. J Ethnopharmacol. 2012; 140 (3): 513–518

[42] Moreira DL, Teixeira SS, Helena MD, Monteiro AC, De-Oliveira ACAX, Paumgartten FJR. Traditional use and safety of herbal medicines. Rev Bras Farmacogn. 2014; 24 (2): 248–257. http://dx.doi.org/10.1016/j.bjp.2014.03.006.

[43] Mussema Y. A historical overview of traditional medicine practices and policy in Ethiopia. Ethiop J Health Dev. 2006; 20 (2): 127–134.

[44] Gedif T, Hahn HJ. The use of medicinal plants in self-care in rural central Ethiopia. J Ethnopharmacol. 2003; 87: 155–161.

[45] Fakeye TO, Adisa R, Musa IE. Attitude and use of herbal medicines among pregnant women in Nigeria. BMC Comp Alternat Med. 2009; 9: 53. DOI: 10.1186/1472-6882-9-53

[46] Bodeker G, Kronenberg F. A public health agenda for traditional, complementary, and alternative medicine. Am J Public Health. 2002; 92 (10): 1582–1591.

[47] Birhan W, Giday W, Teklehemnot T. The contribution of traditional healers' clinic to healthcare system in Adis Ababa, Ethiopia. A cross sectional study. J Ehnobiol Ehthno Med. 7: 23. DOI: 10.1186/1746-4269-7-39

[48] Guo S, DiPietro LA. Factors affecting wound healing. J Dent Res. 2010; 89 (3): 219–229.

[49] Lusby PE, Coombes AL, Wilkinson JM. Bacterial activity of different honeys against pathogenic bacteria. Arch Med Res. 2005; 36: 464–467.

[50] Sarabahi S. Recent advances in topical wound care. Indian J Plast Surg. 2012; 45 (2): 379–387. DOI:10.4103/0970-0358.101321. PMC 3495389.PMID 23162238.

[51] Thakur R, Jain N, Pathak R, Sandhu SS. Practices in wound healing studies of plants. Evid Comp Alternat Med. 2011. DOI:10.1155/2011/438056

[52] White P. The concept of diseases and health care in African traditional religion in Ghana. HTS Teologiese Studies/Theol Stud. 2015; 71 (3). http://dx.doi.org/10.4102/hts.v71i3.2762

[53] Robins H. Culture and wounds. Wound Heal S Afr. 2009; 2 (1): 06–07.

[54] World Health Organization. General guidelines for methodologies on research and evaluation of traditional medicine. 2000; WHO/EDM/TRM/2000. http://apps.who.int/iris/bitstream/10665/66783/1/WHO_EDM_TRM_2000.1.pdf.

[55] Finch C. A new framework for research leading to sports injury prevention. J Sci Med Sport. 2006; 9 (1–2): 3–9.

[56] Atawodi SE, Atawodi JC, Idakwo GA, Pfundstein B, Haubner R, Wurtele G, Bartsch H, Owen RW. Evaluation of the polyphenol content and antioxidant properties of methanol extracts of the leaves, stem, and root barks of *Moringa oleifera* Lam. J Med Food. 2010; 13 (3): 710–716. DOI: 10.1089/jmf.2009.0057.

[57] Juríková T, Mlček J, Sochor J, Hegedűsová A. Polyphenols and their mechanism of action in allergic immune response. Glob J Allergy. 2015; 1 (2): 037–039. DOI: 10.17352/2455-8141.000008

[58] Kanda T, Akiyama H, Yanagida A, Tanabe M, Goda Y, Toyoda M, Teshima R, Saito Y. Inhibitory effects of apple polyphenol on induced histamine release from RBL-2H3 cells and rat mast cells. Biosci Biotechnol Biochem. 1998; 62 (7): 1284–1289.

[59] Tokura T, Nakano N, Ito T, Matsuda H, Nagasako-Akazome Y, Kanda T, Ikeda M, Okumura K, Ogawa H,Nishiyama C. Inhibitory effect of polyphenol-enriched apple extracts on mast cell degranulation *in vitro* targeting the binding between IgE and Fcepsilon RI. Biosci Biotechnol Biochem. 2005; 9 (10): 1974–1977.

[60] Mullen W, Marks SC, Crozier A. Evaluation of phenolic compounds in commercial fruit juices and fruit drinks. J Agric Food Chem. 2007. http://life.umd.edu/classroom/bsci493/Juices.pdf

[61] Guthrie HC, Martin KR, Taylor C, Spear AM, Whiting R, Macildowie S, Clasper JC, Watts SA. A pre-clinical evaluation of silver, iodine and Manuka honey based dressings in a model of traumatic extremity wounds contaminated with *Staphylococcus aureus*. Injury. 2014; 45 (8): 1171–1178DOI: 10.1016/j.injury.2014.05.007. Epub 2014 May 17.

[62] Crane E. Honey from honeybees and other insects. Ethol Ecol Evol. 1991; 3 (1): 100–105. DOI: 10.1080/03949370.1991.10721919

[63] Aparna AR, Rajalakshmi D. Honey-its characteristics, sensory aspects, and applications. Food Rev Int. 1999; 15 (4): 455–471

[64] Mandal MD, Mandal S. Honey: its medicinal property and antibacterial activity. Asian Pac J Trop Biomed. 2011; 1 (2): 154–160.

[65] Hadagali MD, Chua LS. The anti-inflammatory and wound healing properties of honey. Eur Food Res Tech. 2014; 239 (6): 1003–1014.

[66] Wallace E. Feeding the wound: nutrition and wound care. Br J Nurs. 1994; 14–27; 3 (13): 662–667.

[67] Posthauer ME. Nutrition and wound care. Adv Skin Wound Care. 2012; 25 (2): 62–63. DOI: 10.1097/01.ASW.0000411404.19016.ad

[68] Demling RH. Nutrition, anabolism and the wound healing process: an overview. Open Access J Plast Surg. 2009. http://www.ncbi.nlm.nih.gov/pmc/articles/PMC2642618/.

[69] Cerra FB, Lehmann S, Konstantinides N, Dzik J, Fish J, Konstantinides F, LiCari JJ, Holman RT. Improvement in immune function in ICU patients by enteral nutrition supplementation with arginine, RNA, and menhaden oil is independent of nitrogen balance. Nutrition. 1991; 7: 193–199.

[70] Ord H. Nutritional support for patients with infected wounds. Br J Nurs. 2007; 16 (21): 1346–1348, 1350–1352.

[71] Breslow RA, Hallfrisch J, Guy DG, Crawley B, Goldberg AP. The importance of dietary protein in healing pressure ulcers. J Am Geriatr Soc. 1993; 41 (4): 357–362.

[72] Barbul AM. Nutrition and wound healing. Plast Reconstr Surg. 2006; 117 (7 Suppl): 42S–58S.

[73] Nirgiotis JG, Hennessey PJ, Black CT, Andrassy RJ. Low-fat, high-carbohydrate diets improve wound healing and increase protein levels in surgically stressed rats. J Pediatr Surg. 1991; 26 (8): 925–928; Discussion 928–9.

[74] Williams JZ, Barbul A. Nutrition and wound healing. Surg Clin North Am. 2003; 83 (3): 571–596.

[75] Black J, Baharestani MM, Cuddigan J, Dorner B, Edsberg L, Langemo D, et al. National pressure ulcer advisory panel's updated pressure ulcer staging system. Adv Skin Wound Care. 2007; 20 (5): 269–274.

[76] Edmonds J. Nutrition and wound healing: putting theory into practice. Br J Community Nurs. 2007; 12 (12): S31–S34.

[77] Kazembe TC, Gapu P, Duri ZJ. Metals and metal ions in sme plants used for wound healing in Zimbabwe. Bull Environ Pharmacol Life Sci. 2012; 1 (5): 30–39.

[78] AbouZid SF, Mohamed AA. Survey on medicinal plants and spices used in Beni-Sueif, upper Egypt. J Ethnobiol Ethnomed. 2011; 7: 18. DOI: 10.1186/1746-4269-7-18.

[79] Teklehaymanot T, Giday M. Ethnobotanical study of medicinal plants used by people in Zegie Peninsula, northwestern Ethiopia. J Ethnobiol Ethnomed. 2007; 3(12). DOI: 10.1186/1746-4269-3-12.

[80] Inngjerdingen K, Nergård CS, Diallo D, Mounkoro PP, Paulsen BS. An ethnopharmacological survey of plants used for wound healing in Dogonland, Mali, West Africa. J Ethnopharmacol. 2004; 92: 233–244.

[81] Bele MY, Focho DA, Egbe EA, Chuyong BG. Ethnobotanical survey of the uses of Annonaceae around mount Cameroon. Afr J Plt Sci. 2011; 5 (4): 237–247.

[82] Chekole G, Asfaw Z and Kelbessa E. Ethnobotanical study of medicinal plants in the environs of Tara-gedam and Amba remnant forests of Libo Kemkem district, northwest Ethiopia. J Ethnobiol Ethnomed. 2015; 11 4: 1–38. DOI: 10.1186/1746-4269-11-4

[83] Agyarea C, Asaseb A, Lechtenbergc M, Niehuesc M, Detersc A, Henselc A. An ethnopharmacological survey and *in vitro* confirmation of ethnopharmacological use of medicinal plants used for wound healing in Bosomtwi-Atwima-Kwanwoma area, Ghana. J Ethnopharmacol. 2009; 125: 393–403.

[84] Adetutu A, Morgan WA, Corcoran O. Ethnopharmacological survey and *in vitro* evaluation of wound-healing plants used in southwestern Nigeria, J Ethnopharmacol. 2011; 137 (1): 50–56.

[85] Pereira RF, Barrias CC, Granja PL, Bartolo PJ. Advanced biofabrication strategies for skin regeneration and repair. Nanomedicine (Lond). 2013; 8 (4): 603–621. DOI: 10.2217/nnm.13.50

[86] Mensah AY, Houghton PJ, Dickson RA, Fleischer TC, Heinrich M, Bremner P. *In vitro* evaluation of effects of two Ghanaian plants relevant to wound healing. Phytother Res. 2006; 20(11): 941–944.

[87] Annan K, Houghton PJ. Antibacterial, antioxidant and fibroblast growth stimulation of aqueous extracts of *Ficus asperifolia* Miq. and *Gossypiumarboreum* L., wound-healing plants of Ghana, J Ethnopharmacol. 2008; 119: 141–144.

[88] Barku VYA, Opoku-Boahen Y, Owusu-Ansah E, Dayie NTKD, Mensah FE. In-vitro assessment of antioxidant and antimicrobial activities of methanol extracts of six wound healing medicinal plants. J Nat Sci Res. 2013; 3(1): 74–80.

[89] Odukoya OA, Sofidiya MO, Samuel AT, Ajose A, Onalo M, Shuaib B. Documentation of wound healing plants in Lagos-Nigeria: inhibition of lipid peroxidation as in-vivo prognostic biomarkers of activity. Anns Biol Res. 2012; 3(4): 1683–1789.

[90] Adeloye OA, Akinpelu AD, Ogundaini OA, Biodun and Obafemi AC. Studies on antimicrobial, antioxidant and phytochemical analysis of *Urena lobata* leave extract. J Phys Nat Sci. 2007; 1(2): 1–9http://www.scientificjournals.org/journals2007/articles/1281.pdf.

[91] Le NH, Malterud KE, Diallo D, Paulsen BS, Nergård CS, Wangensteen H. Bioactive polyphenols in *Ximenia americana* and the traditional use among Malian healers. J Ethnopharmacol. 2012; 139(3): 858–862.

[92] Aziz DM, Wsoo MA, Ibrahim BM. Antimicrobial and antioxidant activities of extracts from medicinal plant ginger (*Zingiber officinale*) and identification of components by gas chromatography. Afr J Plant Sci. 2015; 9 (10): 412–420.

Chapter 2

Research in Phyto-Constituents for Treatment of Wounds

Chhaya H. Gadgoli

Additional information is available at the end of the chapter

http://dx.doi.org/10.5772/65485

Abstract

Disruption of normal architecture of skin is referred to as wound. There are different types of wounds like contusion, excision, incision, burn, diabetic, etc. The body has its own mechanism to heal wounds in three major overlapping phases, namely inflammatory, proliferative and remodelling. Any agent that promotes the healing process can be utilized as a wound healing agent. Plants have been a great source of medicines to treat wounds. Elucidation of the mechanism of wound healing helped researchers to investigate plants in detail and find out their active constituents. Various biochemical changes take place during the wound healing process, and these changes served as targets for *in vitro* and *in vivo* models. *In vitro* and *in vivo* models are extensively utilized to evaluate wound healing activity. The present chapter gives an overview of some classes of phyto-constituents having wound healing activity.

Keywords: phyto-constitutents, wound healing, models, phases wound healing, mechanism wound healing, treatments of wounds

1. Introduction

The term wound generally refers to the disruption in the normal architecture of skin, which forms the outer protective layer and the largest organ of the integumentary system for all animals and human beings. The skin plays a critical role in fluid homeostasis and provides sensory functions and thermal regulation. About 15–20% of the total body weight composed of skin, and it receives approximately one-third of body's blood supply at the rate of 300 ml/min.

Three main factors can cause injuries to skin and thereby leading to wounds. These factors include environmental, mechanical and chemical. The environmental factors include wind, temperature irregularities, humidity and sunlight. Mechanical injuries may result due to friction, shear force, pressure and epidermal stripping. The chemical injuries are caused by certain irritant chemical substances like corrosive acids, phenols, etc. [1].

Wounds are classified into three major categories, namely open, closed and burn. When the skin is torn, cut or punctured, it is categorized as open while closed wounds involve contusion caused by blunt force trauma. Burn wounds are due to exposure or contact with fire, heat, radiation, chemicals, sunlight, electricity, etc. The tissue injury or wound can follow the mechanism of normal repair, excessive healing or deficient healing depending on physiological, pathological, environmental and nutritional conditions. The normal repair or healing of wounds follows a predictable overlapping phases of inflammation, wound contraction, re-epithelization, tissue remodelling and angiogenesis with granulation tissue formation, in timely manner. The excessive wound healing process leads to the formation of scars, such as keloid. Sometimes, the wound healing process does not progress in the predictive and timely manner leading to impairment of the healing process, and these conditions lead to chronic wounds like venous ulcer.

2. Mechanism of wound healing

Wound healing takes place in four overlapping phases. These involve dynamic and interactive events with involvement of soluble mediators, blood cells, extracellular matrix and parenchymatous cells leading to the restoration of functional and anatomical integrity of skin. The phases of wound healing include inflammatory, proliferative, re-epithelization and remodelling [2, 3]. The cellular and biochemical aspects of these phases are discussed below.

2.1. The inflammatory phase

This phase initiates wound healing cascade and the duration is for about 1–5 days after injury. The phase plays a vital role of clearing the debris and preparation of wound for regeneration of new tissue. Immediately after wounding, within 5–10 minutes, local vasoconstriction takes place and simultaneously the platelets aggregate leading to fibrin clot formation via activation of the coagulation process and release inflammatory cytokines and growth factors. The fibrin clot acts as a matrix for migration of inflammatory cells and is directed to the wound site via chemotaxis from the growth factors such as platelet derived growth factor (PDGF), transforming growth factor-α (TGF-α) and adhesive glycoprotein fibronectin [4]. The brief period of vasoconstriction leads to ischemia of the surrounding tissue. This is followed by sustained vasodilation, in turn increased vascular permeability and migration of neutrophils to the wounded area. Enzymes, fluids and proteins are trapped in the extracellular space leading to inflammation.

This phase is also characterized by oxidative stress as the concentration of reactive oxygen species (ROS) increase. The reactive oxygen species have bacterio-static properties; however, very high concentration of ROS and if the inflammatory conditions are sustained, these can lead to impairment of wound healing [5].

The migration of neutrophils and monocytes to the wound site is also accompanied by mast cells and chemotactic factors released within the 24 hours of injury. The monocyte specific chemotactic factors includes monocyte chemo attractant protein-1 and macrophage inflammatory protein-1. The other chemotactic factors generated during the coagulation stage include kellikerin, fibrinopeptide and fibrin degradation products. Tumour necrosis factor, histamine, cytokines such as interleukin, leukotrienes and proteases represent the inflammatory mediators that are released by mast cells. These serve to up-regulate the intercellular adhesion molecules both on leucocytes and endothelial cell surface through mediating inflammatory cell migration. This results in co-ordination of cell-cell and cell-matrix interactions and thus allowing neutrophils to perform their function of phagocytosis and invasion of microbes.

Proteases such as neutrophil elastase, neutrophil collagenase, known as matrix metalloproteinases (MMPs)-8, are released during the phagocytosis by leucocytes. The proteases initiate wound healing by removing damaged extracellular matrix components and these are replaced by new, intact extra cellular matrix components. The tumour necrosis factor and interleukin 1β, secreted by macrophages, stimulate endothelial cells of capillaries to express cell adhesion molecules and also induce production of cytokine and interleukin-8. These adhesion molecules enable the inflammatory cells to bind to vascular endothelial cells and traverse the capillary basement membrane to enter the surrounding tissues. The tumour necrosis factor also induces the macrophages to produce interleukin-1β and up-regulate MMP expression. Thus, both tumour necrosis factor-β and interleukin-1β directly influence deposition of collagen in wound through inducing collagen synthesis by fibroblasts. The cytokines downregulate expression of tissue inhibitors of MMPs. Macrophages release the angiogenic factor and a growth factor. The growth factor stimulates the fibroblasts production and collagen synthesis in the second phase of wound healing [6].

2.2. The proliferative phase

This phase occurs between days 3–12 after wounding. This is also termed as the granulation phase as it involves proliferation of fibroblast deposition of collagen and other extracellular matrix along with development of new blood vessels.

Cytokines derived from inflammatory cells and epithelial cells regulate the process of cellular migration and proliferation. Various growth factors include insulin like growth factor, basic fibroblast growth factor (bfGF), transforming growth factor (TGF)-β, PDGF and keratinocyte growth factor by fibroblast while TGF-β, TGF-β and interleukin (IL)-1β are synthesized by keratinocytes. Endothelial cells produce vascular endothelial growth factor, bfGF and PDGF. All these mediators are responsible for cell proliferation, synthesis of extracellular matrix proteins and capillary formation. If wound is not infected, the number of inflammatory cells decreases and the fibroblasts along with other cells migrate to the site of wound and proliferate. Fibroblasts get attached to the provisional fibrin matrix and start producing collagen [7–9].

The stages of biosynthesis of collagen include formation of pro-collagen chains, hydroxylation of proline and lysine further extracellular modifications take place leading to deposition and cross linking for formation of the extracellular matrix. Collagen gets its strength in the cross linking step.

2.3. Re-epithelization

This phase includes mitosis of epithelial cells at the wound margin and it begins 24 hours after the injury. The re-epithelization is stimulated by growth factors namely epidermal growth factor (EGF) and TGF-α secreted by the activated macrophages present in wounds. The epithelial cells now start covering the wound area and after completion of complete overlap of the wound area, enzymes are released to dissolve the attachment at the base of scab in turn its removal. Epithelial cell migration needs development of actin filaments within the cytoplasm of the migratory cells and disappearance of desmosomes, which link them to one another and to the basement membrane, respectively. If epidermal basement layer is intact, cells simply migrate over it, however in case of destroyed epidermal basement layer cells initially migrate over the provisional fibrin-fibronectin matrix. As these migrate across the matrix, the epithelial cells regenerate a new basement membrane [10].

2.4. Neoangiogenesis

Various high metabolic activities take place in the wound healing process; hence, there is great demand for oxygen and nutrients. Reduced pH due to the production of lactates and reduced oxygen levels initiate mediators leading to the formation of new blood vessels/capillaries. These are formed as a bud-like structure from pre-existing vessels adjacent to the wound. The new capillaries grow into red loops of blood vessels and give a granular appearance to the wound surface [11–13].

2.5. Remodelling phase

The final stage of wound healing involves formation of an immature collagen matrix into the scar tissue. The new collagen leads to an increase in the tensile strength of skin; however, the strength will be till 80–90% of the original tensile strength. After the formation of initial scar, there is a cessation of proliferation and neo-vascularization, and the remodelling phase begins in the wound. Matrix metalloproteinases secreted by fibroblasts degrade the matrix, and fibronectin gradually disappears and replaces the hyaluronic acid and other amino glycosides by proteoglycans. Proteoglycans are components of the extra cellular matrix, which play an important role in modulating the structure and functions of skin. Proteoglycans impart mechanical strength by their capacity to absorb water and fill the space between the collagen and elastin fibres and also influence collagen formation, cell proliferation, cell migration and cell adhesion during the wound healing process.

Fibroblasts also secrete lysyl oxidase that cross links components of extracellular matrix (ECM). As the scar matures, the angiogenesis decreases; thus, a decrease in the metabolic activin is observed at the wound site and elimination of fibroblasts and macrophages takes place through apoptosis [14, 15].

Human body or animal body has its own capacity to repair the damage occurred to skin with its own pace, however any agent that promotes the process of regeneration can be termed to have wound healing potential. Clinically the main agents used for treatment of wounds include antibiotics to prevent infection and some bio-molecules like collagen. Another source of wound healing agents is plant sources. Many plants have been utilized for treatment of wounds in traditional and folklore medicines. The molecules or the plant as whole or extracts thereof have multiple mechanisms in the regeneration of the skin in injuries. Many such plants have been investigated for their potential in promoting the wound healing process. The knowledge of biochemical, cellular changes that occur during various phases of wound healing help in identifying targets for evaluation of wound healing activity by both *in vivo* and *in vitro* techniques.

3. *In vitro* evaluation of wound healing activity

Various targets are identified to develop a target specific drug, which is an agent that inhibits the molecular target, such as MMP inhibitors and protease inhibitors. These targets are central to the disease mechanism of interests. Cellular targets include the cells involved in the process of wound healing, such as keratinocytes, fibroblasts and immune cells.

3.1. Targets of cellular activity

Any agent, which decreases the bleeding time, that is the first stage of wound healing, has the potential to promote wound healing, as these have a positive effect on integrity of blood vessels or active participation of platelets in forming haemostatic plug. The effect of any agent or extract on angiogenesis is studied by Chick Chorioallantoic Membrane Assay (CAM) [16].

The proteases released are helpful as wound diagnostics. Proteases are also known as proteinases, which play a vital role in normal wound healing processes. One of the important families of proteases, matrix metalloproteinases (MMPs), plays an important role in wound healing. These preferentially breakdown proteins comprise of extracellular tissues and require zinc at the active centre of the ion. MMPs are produced by activated inflammatory cells (neutrophils and macrophages) and wound cells (epithelial cells, fibroblasts and vascular endothelial cells). Most of the MMPs are secreted in the extracellular matrix; some are also associated with cell membranes and are known as membrane type MMPs [17].

The important functions of proteases in the inflammatory phase include removal of the damaged extracellular matrix. In phase II of wound healing, that is proliferation stage, proteases degrade the capillary basement membrane to promote angiogenesis, and also aid in detachment. MMP-1 is responsible for migration of cells. In the last phase, that is the remodelling phase, proteases are responsible for contraction and remodelling of the scar extracellular matrix. The amounts of proteases are very critical as the excess amount of proteases lead to degradation of the newly formed extracellular matrix and growth factors leading to delayed wound healing. MMP-9 has shown inverse correlation with the wound healing process and the most non-healing wounds are found to have high levels of MMP-9 [18]. The levels of inflammatory markers, high levels of proteases including MMPs, and diminished growth factor activity can be treated as markers of the wound healing process [19, 20].

3.2. Skin cells: targets for wound healing

Fibroblasts are the key players in the process of wound healing through contraction, synthesis and deposition of the extracellular matrix; hence, the fibroblast *in vitro* model is apt to correlate contractile events of wound healing. *In vitro* fibroblast bioassay involves isolation of human dermal fibroblasts from post auricular surgery, followed by culturing in laboratories. These fibroblast cultures are then incubated with the test substances, and the content of hydroxyproline/100 mg of DNA is estimated [21].

Keratinocytes assay involves isolation of keratinocytes from human foreskin or residual skin samples removed during surgery, followed by culturing in laboratories. Wound is inflicted in the culture through gentle scrapping. The cells are then incubated with the test sample. The effect of test sample on proliferation and motility of keratinocytes is studied. The greater the proliferation and motility as compared to the untreated cells indicate the promotion of the wound healing process [22].

4. *In vivo* models for wound healing

The *in vivo* studies are generally carried out in animals like mice, rats, guinea pigs, through inflicting wounds of various types like excision, incision, burn, dead space, diabetic wounds, etc. The most popularly studied wound models include excision, incision and dead space. The general method of evaluation of any test substance for its wound healing potential includes evaluation of acute dermal toxicity of the base utilized for preparation of topical preparation and the test substance in its highest concentration that would be incorporated into the base. The acute dermal toxicity is evaluated in animals like albino rats using the protocols described in OECD Guidelines number 434. Once the substance and the base is proved to be safe, it is then evaluated using the following standard models.

The animals are divided into three main groups, namely control indicating the normal wound healing mechanism of body without any treatment, vehicle control is treated with the base only and the test group is treated with the test substance(s).

4.1. Excision wound model

The animals utilized for wound healing studies are depilated on their thoracic region and excision wounds are inflicted on the thoracic region using sharp gadgets covering an area of about 500 mm^2 and a depth of about 2 mm (**Figure 1**). The wounds are cleaned using cotton swab and are treated most of the time topically but it is also observed that sometimes studies are carried out by oral treatment with the test substance. The day of infliction of wound is considered as zero and the area of the wound is traced on an OHP sheet. The percentage wound closure is determined by tracing the wound on alternative days and calculating the area of wound. The results of the test substances are compared with the untreated or vehicle treated wounds. The reduction in the number of days for closing the wounds as compared to the untreated wound indicates the promotion of the wound healing process [23]. The progress of healing of wound is also monitored by period of epithelization, histological studies and estimation of biochemical parameters like hydroxyproline, hexosamine, collagen content in granulation tissue on day 11 after wounding [24–26].

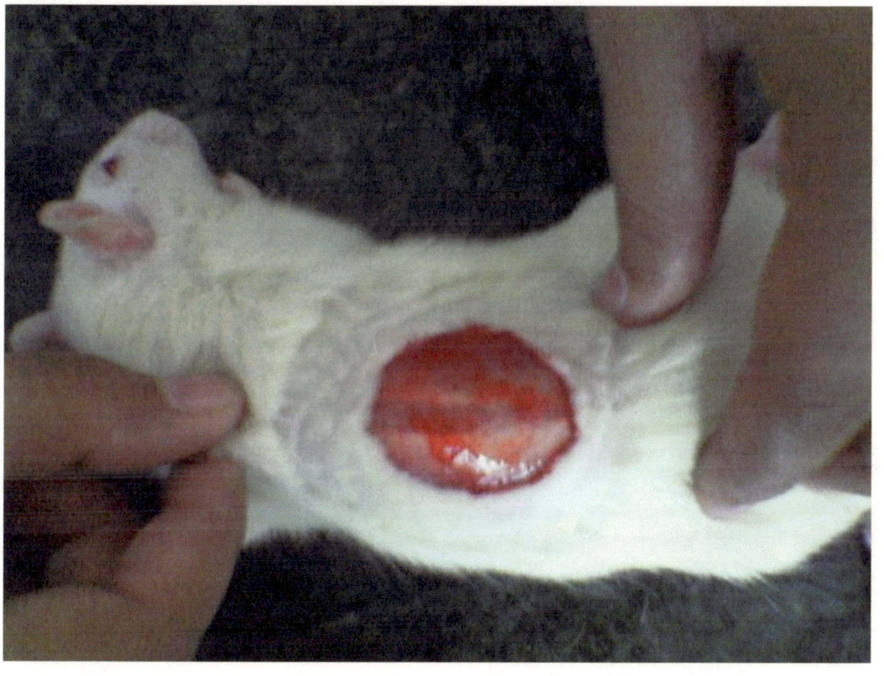

Figure 1. Excision wound inflicted in the thoracic region of the albino rat.

4.2. Incision wound model

The model simulates surgical wounds. These are inflicted by giving longitudinal paravertebral incisions through the skin and cutaneous muscles at a distance of about of about 1.5 cm from midline on either side of the vertebral column. After cleaning of the wound, the parted skin is stitched with interrupted sutures (**Figure 2**). The wounds are treated either locally or orally with the test substance and the stitches are opened on day 10. The tensile strength of the treated skin is measured as a parameter for the repairing of skin [27]. The tensile strength of the repaired skin can be measured by a tensiometer indicated in **Figure 3**, which was constructed in our laboratory. Higher tensile strength of the repaired skin as compared to the untreated skin is an indication of promotion of the wound healing process.

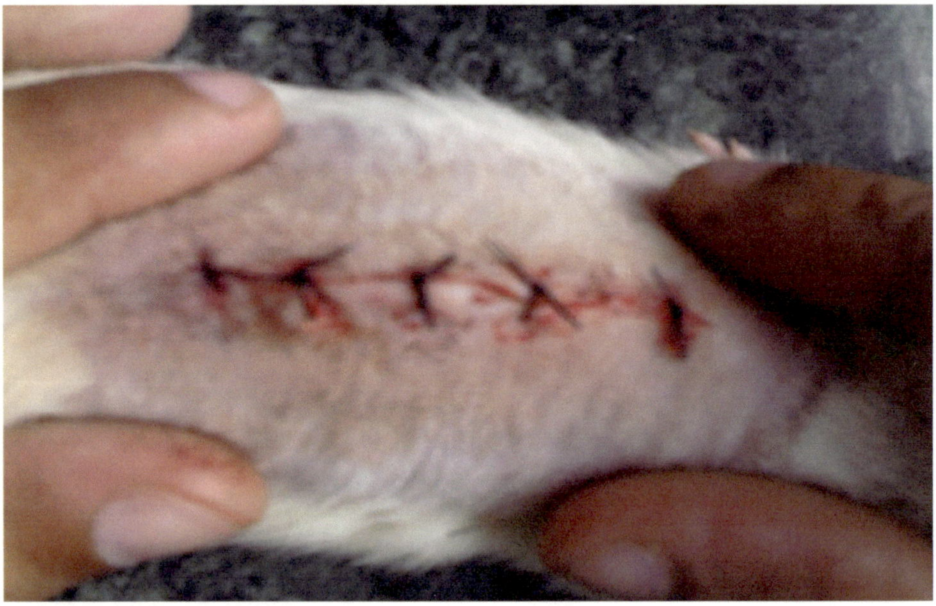

Figure 2. Sutured incision wound inflicted on the back of the albino rat.

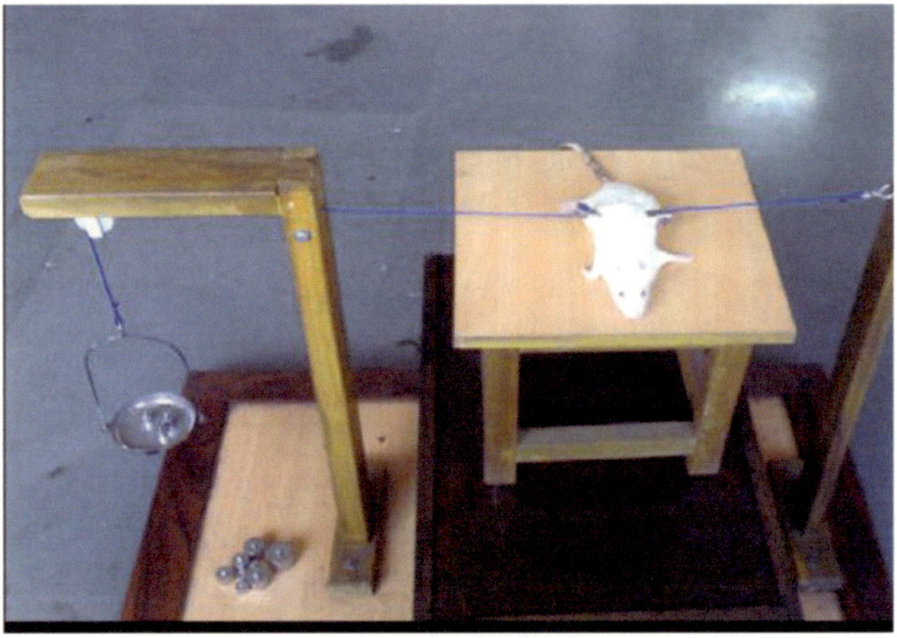

Figure 3. Tensiometer for determination of tensile strength of repaired skin of the albino rat.

4.3. Dead space wound model

The model is useful to study physical and mechanical changes in granulation tissue. In this model, subcutaneous dead space wounds are inflicted on either side of axilla and groin on the ventral surface of animal by creating a pouch through a small nick in skin followed by insertion of a sterile cylindrical object made up of glass or polypropylene or sterile cotton pallet in the pouch. The wounds are then sutured and treated with the test substance either locally or orally for 10 days [28]. The objects inserted are taken out through surgical procedures and the physical changes in the granuloma tissues are studied along with the determination of biochemical markers, like hydroxyl proline, hexosamine, etc.

Histopathological studies on the granulation tissue also reveal the extent of healing. Sections of granulation tissue are formed during the healing process [29].

4.4. Burn wound model

Burn wounds are inflicted using heated gadgets like hot metal cylinder, metal plate or using hot molten wax [30]. Promotion of healing by the test substance is monitored in the same way as described in the excision wound model.

5. Phyto-constituents with wound healing activity

Plants have been used in many traditional systems of medicine for healing wounds. With the advent of elucidation of the mechanism of wound healing at cellular and molecular levels and based on the knowledge of various plants used in traditional systems of medicines for treatment of wounds, scientific investigations were triggered to get agents/drugs for healing wounds. There is another major reason for the research in wound healing agents, is non-availability of specific wound healing agents, except the use of antibiotics, anti-inflammatory and analgesic drugs in the allopathic system of medicines.

Plants are a good source of chemically diverse phyto-constituents and these are assimilated by human and animal bodies easily as compared to the synthetic molecules and hence render a pharmacophore for the development of drugs. Several papers have been published indicating the investigation of plant extracts for their potential as wound healing agents, however very few plants have been investigated in detail explaining the constituents responsible and the mechanism of action of wound healing.

Chemically phyto-constituents are classified into major categories like alkaloids, glycosides, terpenoid, quinines, flavonoids, polyphenols, sulphur-containing compounds, polyacetylenes, polyketides and steroids. It is observed that the compounds having anti-inflammatory, antibacterial, astringent, antioxidant activities and immunomodulatory activities, indicated to promote the wound healing process.

5.1. Quinones

Quinones are oxidized derivatives of phenols and catechols. Three types of quinones occur in nature namely Benzo (1,2/1,4), naphtha (1,4) and anthra (9,10). Benzoquinones occurring in nature include embelin (I) from berries of *Embelia ribes* and Co-enzyme Q10 (Co-Q10) (II) which is also known as ubiquinone is a biosynthesized quinone with 10 isoprene side chains in humans. Radhakrishnan et al. [31] in their study on the effect of Co-Q10 Radhakrishnan on cutaneous healing of skin incised mice revealed that the compound has antioxidant activity in which it is converted to reduced (CoQ10H) in the presence of some kinds of intracellular reducing agents and it has increased levels of collagen-like polymer in the granulation tissue of animals.

Embelin is a well-known anthelmintic agent and also reported to have antibacterial activity and wound healing activity [32]. Incision wound treated with embelin indicated a higher rate of wound contraction and tensile strength with increased cross linking of collagen fibres was observed in granulation tissues as compared to the standard skin ointment, Framycetin. Embelin has structural resemblance to vitamin E that is alpha tocopherol (III) which is a well-known antioxidant. Lin et al. [33] studied the effect of application of topical tocopherol cream on cutaneous wound healing in Streptozotocin-induced diabetic rats. It was revealed that the cream containing 0.29% w/w of tocopherol could promote healing of the excision wounds in diabetic rats.

Many naphthaquinone derivatives found in plants have been observed to possess wound healing activity. The popular one include alkannins and shikonins [34]. Alkannins and shikonins (IV a & b) are chiral-pairs of naturally occurring isohexenylnaphthazarins. They are found in the external layer of the roots of at least a hundred and fifty species that belong mainly to the genera *Alkanna, Lithospermum, Echium, Onosma* and *Arnebia* of the Boraginaceae family. The alkannin, shikonin and their derivatives possess potent antimicrobial and anti-inflammatory properties and are revealed to actively support the proliferative phase of wound healing. Papageorgiou et al. [35, 36] isolated alkannin, shikonin and derivatives to be active constituents from roots of Boraginaceae family and carried out clinical studies on alkannins and shikonins for treatment of non-healing venous wounds and reported the molecules could effectively heal the wounds. Dimer of naphthaquinone (V) [37] was isolated and the structure of the same was elucidated by Gawand et al. and reported it to be active wound healing agent through animal studies. Lawsone (VI) obtained from Leaves of *Lawsonia alba* and *L. inermis* was complexed with zinc and the wound healing activity of the complex [38] was evaluated using excision and incision wound models. The complex indicated good antimicrobial activity and displayed to promote the proliferative phase.

One of the anthraquinone derivatives Emodin (VII) [1,3,8– trihydroxy—6–methyl anthraquinone] obtained from rhizomes of, is reported to promote the repair of excision wounds in animals via a complex mechanism involving stimulation of tissue regeneration and regulating Smad-mediated TGF-beta(1) signalling pathway [39].

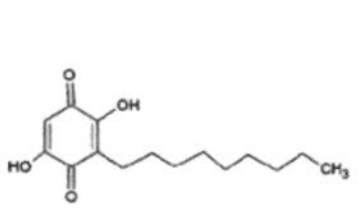
(I)

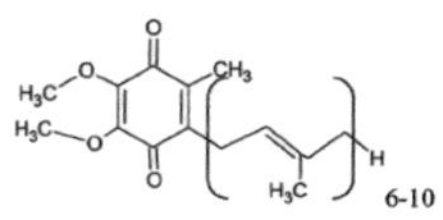
(II)

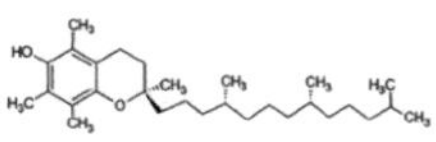
(III)

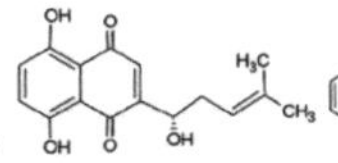
(IVa)

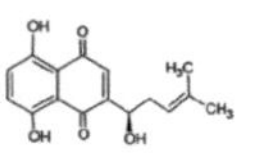
(IVb)

V – OE1

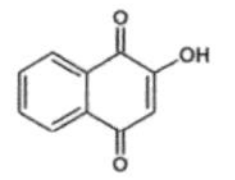
(VI)

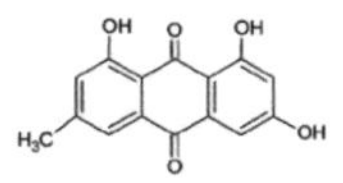
(VII)

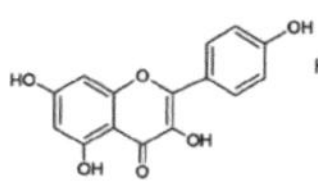
(IX)

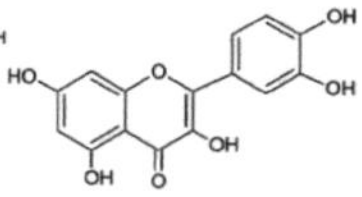
(X)

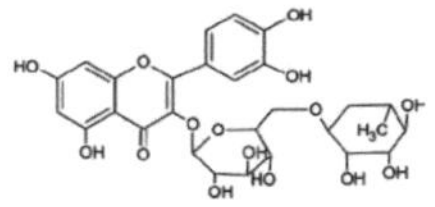
(XI)

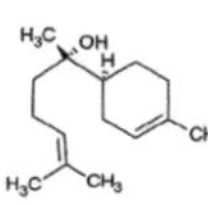
XII a

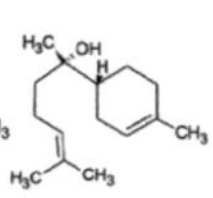
XIIb

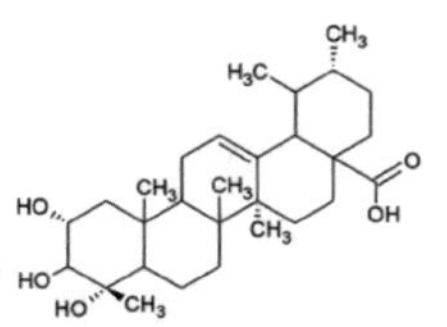
XIII

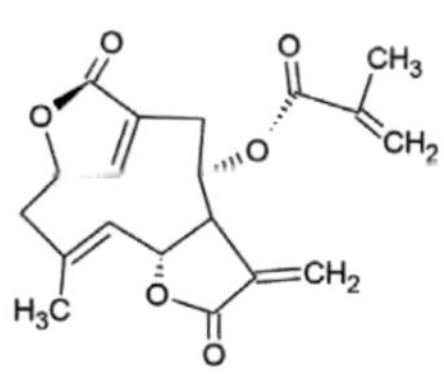
(XIV)

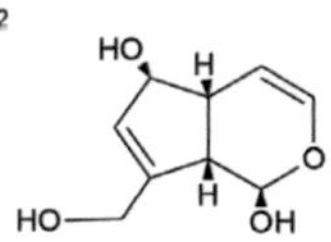
(XV)

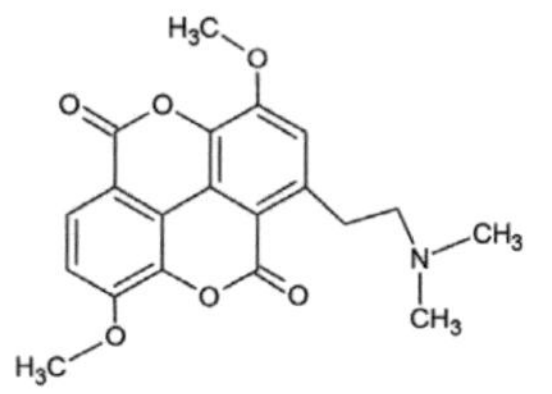
(XVI)

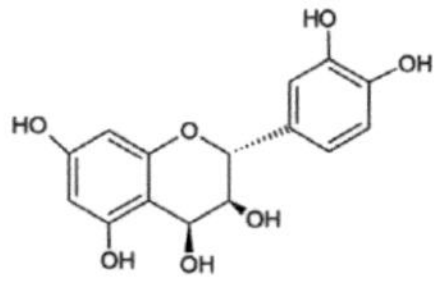
(XVII)

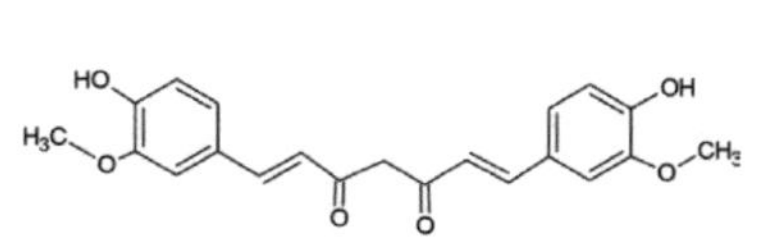
(XVIII)

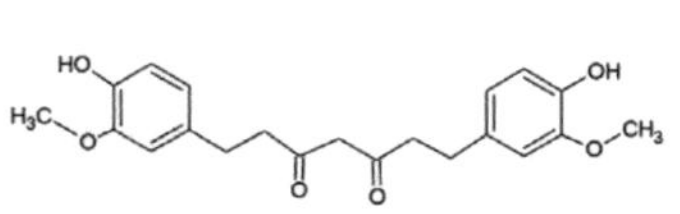
(XIX)

5.2. Phenolics and polyphenolics

Phenolic compounds include simple phenolic compounds, phenyl propanoids, lignans, lignins, flavonoids and polyphenols include tannins. Tannins have mainly antibacterial, antioxidants and astringent activities. Phenyl propanoid glycosides namely verbascoside and teopolioside are structurally characterized to contain caffeic acid and 4,5-hydroxyl ethanol [40] were isolated from *Syringa vulgaris* and *Ajuga reptans* plant cell lines, respectively, were studied for wound healing activity by both *in vitro* and *in vivo* techniques. The compounds exhibited good anti-inflammatory, antioxidant and wound healing activities. Both the compounds were extremely effective inhibitors of chemokine and growth factor expression by cultured human keratinocytes treated with pro-inflammatory cytokines, TNF-α and interferon gamma.

Another group of phenolic compounds include flavonoids and these are one of the vast groups of phyto-constituents with large structural diversity. The chemical nuclei of flavonoids described as Benzopyran. Kaempferol (IX) and Quercetin (X) occurring in onion extract are reported [41] to increase type-1 collagen through increased expression of MMP-1, revealing their role in the anti-scar effect in skin. One of the popular flavonoidal glycoside of Quercetin is Rutin (Quercetin-3-o-rutinoside) (XI) commercialized to be administered orally, supported wound healing through enhanced production and accumulation of extracellular matrix. Rutin conjugated hydrogels in wound dressing was found to promote the wound healing process. Anthocyanins are reported to stimulate wound induced VEGF production in fibroblast and keratinocytes, also reduce the adhesion of inflammatory monocytes to endothelial cells [42].

Fruit pulp of *Musa sapientum* exhibited wound healing activity in animals, increased tensile strength, collagen formation which was revealed through the elevated levels of hydroxyproline, hexosamine and the wound contraction rate. Docking studies on Leucocyanidin (XVII) from the fruit indicated inhibition of MMPs, like collagenase, gelatinase, elastase and stromelysine [43].

The astringent property of tannins plays a vital role in wound contraction and increased rate of epithelization in phase three [40]. The tannin extract from *Terminalia arjuna* exhibited angiogenic activity through up-regulating VEGF-A expression in the inflammatory phase [44]. Experiments conducted with tannic acid cross-linked collagen scaffolds demonstrated a significant effect on the wound healing process. The other tannins like proanthocyanidin from grape seed displayed accelerated wound contraction and closure associated with the hyperproliferative epithelial region [45]. Proanthocyanidins are high molecular weight oligomers consisting of 4–11 units of flavan-9-ol. These form complexes with proteins and precipitate them leading to enzyme inhibition involved in vascular tissue degradation [46]. Extracts of grape seed proanthocyanidins are reported to stimulate the expression of VEGF in cultured keratinocytes and thus promote the wound healing process [45, 47].

5.3. Terpenoids

Terpenoids form a broad class of phyto-constituent derived from acetate mevalonic acid pathway. The isoprene (C_5H_8) unit is a monomer for various terpenoids. Based on the number of isoprene units in a molecule decide the type of terpenoid, namely for two isoprene units it is mono-terpene, three isoprene units it is sesquiterpene, four isoprene units it is di-terpene, for four isoprene units it tri-terpene and for eight isoprene units it tetraterepenes or also referred to carotenoids.

Mono-terpenes and sesquiterpenes generally form the major constituents of volatile oils. *Matricaria chamomilla* is popularly used as nutraceutical for its anti-inflammatory activity. The volatile oil of flowers is rich in (+) epi-α-bisabol and its (-)enantiomer (XII a & b). Wound healing studies on the bisabols revealed to shorten the healing period in cutaneous burns of guinea pigs exposed to UV light [48] and the probable mechanism for wound healing activity reported in another study involved increasing cell migration [49]. Asiaticoside (XIII) isolated from *Centella asiatica* was found to increase the rate of wound healing through collagen synthesis in turn increasing tensile strength [50]. An active sesquiterpene lactone deoxyelephantopin (XIV) was isolated from ethanolic extract of leaves of *Elephantopus scaber* by Singh et al. [51] and reported that the presence of alpha methylene gama lactone is an essential structural feature for wound healing activity. The compound exhibited wound healing activity at all the three phases. Carotenoids like retinoids are found to reverse the impaired healing of wound by acting on growth factors and collagen deposition.

Iridoids are classified under the category of mono- terpenoids and occur as glucosides. These are structurally bicyclic cis fused cyclopentane-pyrans and have diverse pharmacological activities like anti-inflammatory, antimicrobial, anti-viral, hepatoprotective, etc. One of the iriod glycosides Aucubin (XV) (0.1% solution) isolated from *Aucuba japonica* was reported to have an anti-inflammatory effect on oral mucosal wound healing, and to promote early re-epithelialization and collagen matrix formation [52].

5.4. Alkaloids

Alkaloids form one of the vast categories of phyto-constituents. These are basic secondary metabolites with presence of nitrogen either in the heterocyclic ring or outside the ring and exhibit marked physiological actions when administered to animals or human beings. These have varied pharmacological actions like anticancer, emetic, hypotensive, etc. One of the well investigated alkaloids is Tapsine (XVI) obtained from *Croton lechleri* (*Euphorbiaceae*) is found to be potent wound healing agent as earlier phases of wound healing presumably by increasing the migration of fibroblasts to the wounded area [49, 53]. Aconite alkaloids exhibited wound healing activity through stimulation of growth of colonies from fibroblasts precursors [54, 55].

5.5. Steroids

Steroids are non-polar secondary metabolites and are described to possess a cyclopentano-perhydrophenanthrene nucleus. These are biosynthesized through the acetate mevalonic acid pathway. Stigmastatone was isolated from bark of *Celastrus paniculatus* and was studied for enzyme target glycogen synthase kinase-3-β (GSK-3-β), an important regulatory enzyme whose inhibition promotes wound healing through β-catanin dependent Wnt signalling pathway. The molecule was docked with GSK-3-β, and it was observed that the molecule leads to the inhibition of the enzyme with an IC_{50} value of 1.21 Nm while nitrofurazone indicated an IC_{50} value of 1.35 nM. Further evaluation of *in vivo* models of excision, incision and dead space wounds, the compound exhibited wound healing activity with increased tensile strength and collagenation of granulation tissue [56].

5.6. Polysaccharides

Aloe species are known for the presence of anthraquinone glycosides and the derivatives are popularly utilized for purgative actions. Aloe species also contain glucomannans which find their applications in the cosmetic industry in moisturising and anti-ageing products. *Aloe vera* is reported to heal second degree burn wounds and this property is attributed to the presence of mannose-6-phosphate. It is also reported that glucomannans interact with growth factor receptors of fibroblasts and stimulate its activity and proliferation in turn increase collagen synthesis when administered by both oral and topical route. Acetylated mannose is also termed as acemannan forms a major component of *Aloe vera* and this accelerates wound healing and also reported to have potential to stimulate release of fibrogenic cytokines [57–60].

A phyto-constituent from the class of arylheptanoids is curcumin (XVIII), a colouring matter obtained from the rhizomes of *Curcuma longa*, a very important molecule as it has array of pharmacological activities. The molecule is very well investigated and lot of research has been envisaged for formulations to improve bioavailability of the molecule. It is a good anti-inflammatory agent and has been used since ages to treat wounds. It is also proved to be good wound healing agent [61, 62].

The mechanism of enhancing the wound healing rate was reported [63] to be through increased cellular proliferation and collagen synthesis. It was observed that there is increase in DNA, total protein and type III collagen in wound tissues. The increased collagen synthesis was also responsible for increased tensile strength of repaired skin. The antioxidant property of collagen also played a vital role in promoting wound healing. The antioxidant property of the molecule was revealed through decreased levels of lipid peroxides and increased levels of superoxide dismutase, catalase and glutathione peroxidase.

Tetrahydrocurcumin (XIX), a metabolite of curcumin, also exhibits many pharmacological actions. The poor bioavailability of the molecule has been overcome by preparation of a water soluble derivative, glycosylated tetrahydrocurcumin. The product has an advantage of being colourless and also increased cutaneous absorption of the molecule thereby exhibiting good wound healing properties [64–66].

6. Conclusion and summary

Currently antibacterial and antibiotics are utilized for treatment of wound. Based on the knowledge of traditional medicines and folklore medicines, many plants have been screened for wound healing activity. Some plants are investigated in detail to get an active wound healing agent; however, very few have reached till clinical use. There is still scope to carry out more research in the area and get molecules with clinical applications. The following chart

http://dx.doi.org/10.5772/65485

indicates the summary of the mechanism of wound healing and various targets, which can be utilized in development of wound healing agent (**Figure 4**).

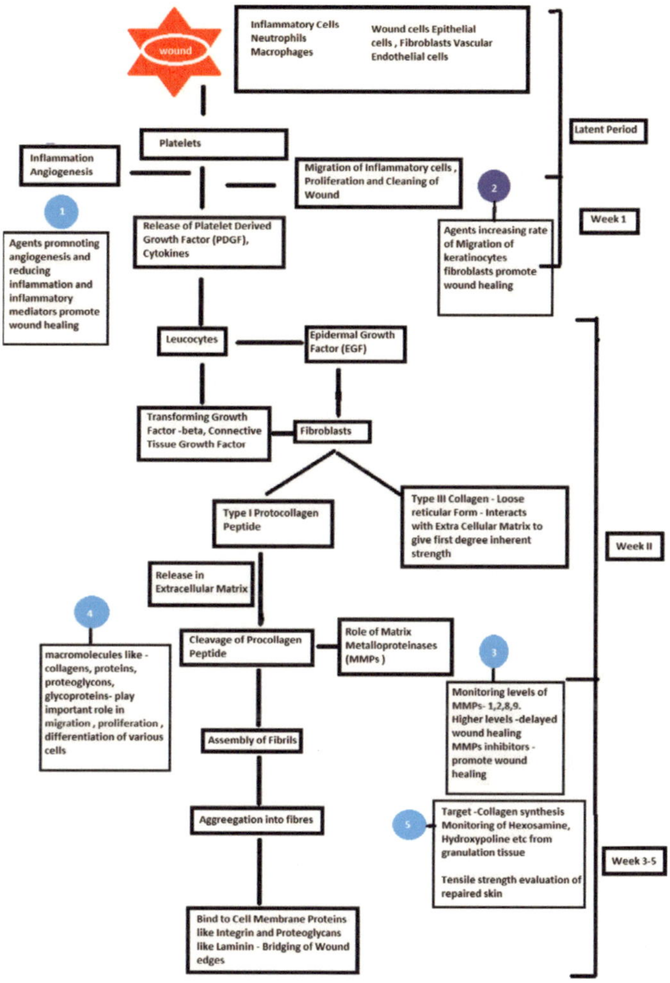

Figure 4. Summary of the mechanism of wound healing and various targets.

Author details

Chhaya H. Gadgoli

Address all correspondence to: chhayahg@rediffmail.com

Saraswathi Vidya Bhavan's College of Pharmacy, Dombivli (E), Maharashtra, India

References

[1] Newfoundland Labrador Skin and Wound Care Manual. 2008: 1–135. Available online: http://westernhealth.nl.ca/uploads/PDFs/wound%20care%20manual%20for%20dianne%20clements%20final.pdf

[2] Saha R. Unseen aspects of wound healing: an overview. International Journal of Pharma and Bio Sciences 2011: 2(4): 275–285.

[3] Singer AJ, Clark RAF. Cutaneous wound healing. The New England Journal of Medicine 1999: 341: 738–746.

[4] Karukonda SRK, Flynn TC, Boh EE, McBurney EI, Russo GG, Millikan LE. The effects of drugs on wound healing – part 2. International Journal of Dermatology 2000: 39(5): 321–333.

[5] Nanney LB, King LE Jr. Epidermal growth factor and transforming growth factor-β, in: *The Molecular and Cellular Biology of Wound Repair* (Clark RAF, ed.), 2nd ed., Plenum, New York, 1996: pp. 171–194.

[6] Bennett NT, Schultz GS. Growth factors and wound healing: biochemical properties of growth factors and their receptors. American Journal of Surgery 1993: 165(6): 728–737.

[7] Li J, Chen J, Kirsner R. Pathophysiology of acute wound healing. Clinics in Dermatology 2007: 25(1): 9–18.

[8] Diegelmann RF, Evans MC. Wound healing: an overview of acute, fibrotic and delayed healing. Frontiers in Bioscience 2004: 9: 283–289.

[9] Battegay EJ. Angiogenesis: mechanistic insights, neovascular diseases, and therapeutic prospects. Journal of Molecular Medicine 1995: 73(7): 333–346.

[10] Monaco JL, Lawrence T. Acute wound healing: an overview. Clinics in Plastic Surgery 2003: 30(1): 1–12.

[11] Jacobi J, Tam BY, Sundram U, von Degenfeld G, Blau HM, Kuo CJ, Cooke JP. Discordant effects of a soluble VEGF receptor on wound healing and angiogenesis. Gene Therapy 2004: 11(3): 302–309.

[12] Barleon B, Sozzani S, Zhou D, Weich HA, Mantovani A, Marme D. Migration of human monocytes in response to vascular endothelial growth factor (VEGF) is mediated via the VEGF receptor flt-1. Blood 1996: 87(8): 3336–3343.

[13] Sawano A, Iwai S, Sakurai Y, et al. Flt-1, vascular endothelial growth factor receptor 1, is a novel cell surface marker for the lineage of monocyte-macrophages in humans. Blood 2001: 97(3): 785–791.

[14] Madden JW, Peacock EE Jr. Studies on the biology of collagen during wound healing. I. Rate of collagen synthesis and deposition in cutaneous wounds of the rat. Surgery 1968: 64: 288–294.

[15] Osterholm C, Barczyk MM, Busse M, Grønning M, Reed RK, Kusche-Gullberg M. Mutation in the heparan sulfate biosynthesis enzyme EXT1 influences growth factor signaling and fibroblast interactions with the extracellular matrix. Journal of Biological Chemistry 2009: 284: 34935–34943.

[16] Chris S, David M, Dwayne G. Stupack angiogenesis assays in the chick CAM. Methods in Molecular Biology 2005: 294: 123–136.

[17] Vartak DG, Gemeinhart RA. Matrix metalloproteinases: underutilized targets for drug delivery. Journal of Drug Targeting 2007: 15(1): 1–20.

[18] Gibson D, Cullen B, Legerstee R, Harding KG, Schultz G. MMPs made easy. Wound International 2009: 1(1): 1–6. Available from http://www.woundsinternational.com

[19] Lam S, van der Geest RN, Verhagen NAM, van Nieuwenhoven FA, Blom IE, Aten J, Goldschmeding R, Daha MR, van Kooten C. Connective tissue growth factor and IGF-I are produced by human renal fibroblasts and cooperate in the induction of collagen production by high glucose. Diabetes 2003: 52(12): 2975–2983.

[20] Rodrigues HG, Vinolo MAR, Magdalon J, Vitzel K, Nachbar RT, Ana Flavia M, Pessoa AFM, dos Santos MF, Hatanaka E, Calder PC, Cur R. Oral administration of oleic or linoleic acid accelerates the inflammatory phase of wound healing. Journal of Investigative Dermatology 2012: 132(1): 208–215.

[21] Houghton PJ, Hylands PJ, Mensah AY, Hensel A, Deters AM. In vitro tests and ethnopharmacological investigations: wound healing as an example. Journal of Ethnopharmacology 2005: 100: 100–107.

[22] Jonkman JEN, Cathcart JA, Feng Xu, Bartolini ME, Amon JE, Katarzyna MS, Colarusso P. Special focus: live imaging: an introduction to the wound healing assay using live-cell microscopy. Cell Adhesion & Migration 2014: 8(5): 440–451.

[23] Davidson JM. Animal models for wound repair. Archives of Dermatological Research 1998: 290(1): S1–S11.

[24] Werner S, Breeden M, Hubner G, Greenhalgh DG, Longaker MT. Induction of keratinocyte growth factor expression is reduced and delayed during wound healing in the genetically diabetic mouse. Journal of Investigation in Dermatology 1994: 103: 469–473.

[25] Bergman I, Loxley R. Two improved and simplified methods for the spectrophotometeric determination of hydroxyproline. Safety in Mine Research Establishment, Ministry of Power, Sheffield, England 1963: 35(12): 1961–1965.

[26] Ehrlich HP, Hunt TK. Effect of cortisone and anabolic steroids on tensile strength of a healing wound. Annals of Surgery 1969: 170: 203–206.

[27] Nath V, Singh M, Govindrajan R, Rawat AKS, Mehrotra S. Antimicrobial, wound healing and antioxidant activity of *Plagiochasma appendiculatum* Lehm. et Lind. Journal of Ethnopharmacology 2006: 107: 67–72.

[28] Choi BS, Song HS, Kim HR, Park TW, Kim TD, Cho BJ, Kim CJ, Sim SS. Effect of coenzyme Q10 on cutaneous healing in skin-incised mice. Archives of Pharmaceutical Research 2009: 32(6): 907–913. doi: 10.1007/s12272-009-1613-3. Epub 2009 Jun 26.

[29] Shenoy RR, Sudheendra AT, Nayak PG, Paul P. Normal and delayed wound healing is improved by sesamol, an active constituent of *Sesamum indicum* Linn. in albino rats. Journal of Ethnopharmacology 2011: 133: 608–612.

[30] Kiyoshi J, Junior M, Gragnani A, Luiza M, Ramos C, Ferreira LM. Rat an experimental model for burns. A systematic review. Acta Cirúrgica Brasileira 2012: 27(6): 417–423.

[31] Radhakrishnan N, Gnanamani A, Mandal AB M A potential antibacterial agent Embelin, a natural benzoquinone extracted from *Embelia ribes* Biology and Medicine, 3 (2) Special Issue: 2011: 1–7, 1 MAASCON–1 (Oct 23–24, 2010): "Frontiers in Life Sciences: Basic and Applied" eISSN: 09748369, www.biolmedonline.com

[32] Swamy HMK, Krishna V, Shankarmurthy K, Rahiman BA, Mankani KL, Mahadevan KM, Harish BG, Naika HR. Wound healing activity of Embeline isolated from ethanol extract of leaves of *Embelia ribes* Burn. Journal of Ethnopharmacology 2007: 109(3): 529–534.

[33] Lin TS, Abd Latiff A, Hamid NAA, Wan Ngah WZ, Mazlan M. Evaluation of topical tocopherol cream on cutaneous wound healing in Streptozotocin-induced diabetic rats. Evidence-Based Complementary and Alternative Medicine 2012: Article ID 491027: 6. http://dx.doi.org/10.1155/2012/491027

[34] Vassilios P, Papageorgiou, AN, Assimopoulou, EA, Couladouros, David H, and Nicolaou KC: The Chemistry and Biology of Alkannin, Shikonin, and Related Naphthazarin Natural Products, Angewandi Chemistry, Int. Ed. 1999: 18: 270–300.

[35] Papageorgiou VP, Assimopoulou AN, Ballis AC. Alkannins and shikonins: a new class of wound healing agents. Current Medicinal Chemistry 2008: 15: 3248–3267.

[36] Mani H, Sidhu GS, Singh AK, Gaddipati J, Banaudha KK, Raj K. and Maheshwari RK. Enhancement of Wound Healing by Shikonin Analogue 93/637 in Normal and Impaired Healing, Skin Pharmacol Physiol 2004:17:49–56 (DOI:10.1159/000074063).

[37] Gawand N, Purnima V and Gadgoli C. Wound healing activity of oligomer of alkanin/ shikonin isolated from root bark of *Onosma echioides.* Natural Product Research 2015: 29(16): 1584–1588.

[38] Gadgoli C, Bandewar P and Waghulde S. Use of Lawsone Complexes for Promoting Wound Healing And As An Antimicrobial Agent. Indian Patent Office No. 2878/MUM/2011, 11/10/2011.

[39] Korkina LG, Mikhal'chik EV, Suprun MV, Pastore S, Dal Toso R. Molecular mechanisms underlying wound healing and anti-inflammatory properties of naturally occurring biotechnologically produced phenylpropanoid glycosides. Cellular and Molecular Biology 2007: 53(5): 84–91. doi: 10.117 /T822

[40] Tang T, Yin L, Yang J, Shan G. Emodin, an anthraquinone derivative from Rheum officinale Baill, enhances cutaneous wound healing in rats. European Journal of Pharmacology 2007: 567(3): 177–185.

[41] Cho JW, Cho SY, Lee SR, Lee KS. Onion extract and Quercetin induce matrix metalloproteinase-1 in-vitro and in-vivo. International Journal of Molecular Medicine 2010: 25(3): 347–352.

[42] Tran NQ, Joung YK, Lih E, Park K. In-situ forming and rutin releasing chitosan hydrogels as injectable dressings for dermal wound healing. Biomacromolecules 2011: 12(8): 2872–2880.

[43] Nizamutdinova IT, Kim YM, Chung JI, Schin SC, Jeong YK, Seo HG, Lee JH, Chang KC, Kim HJ. Anthocyanin from black soyabean seed coats stimulate wound healing in fibroblasts and keratinocytes and prevent inflammation in endothelial cells. Food and Chemical Toxicology 2009: 47(11): 2806–2812.

[44] Singh A, Mishra A, Verma S, Gautam MK, Goel RK. MMPs as molecular targets for wound healing by *Musa sapientum*: *in-silico* and *in-vivo* evidences. Research and reviews. Journal of Pharmacology and Toxicological Studies 2014: 2(1): 39–46.

[45] Chaudhari M, Mengi S. Evaluation of phytoconstitutents of *Terminalia arjuna* for wound healing activity in rats. Phytotherapy Research 2006: 20(9): 799–805.

[46] Li K, Dia Y, Zhang H, Wang S, Zhang Z, Yu B, Huang S, Yang H. Tannin extracts from immature fruits of Terminalia chebula Fructus Retz. promote cutaneous wound healing in rats. BMC Complementary and Alternative Medicine 2011: 11(86): 1–9.

[47] Khanna S, Venojarvi M, Roy S, Sharma N, Trikha P, Bagchi D, Bagchi M, Sen CK. Dermal wound healing properties of redox-active grape seed proanthocyanidins. Free Radical Biological Medicine 2002: 33: 1089–1096.

[48] Baxter NJ, Lilley TH, Haslam E, Williamson MP. Multiple interactions between polyphenols and a salivary proline-rich protein repeat result in complexation and precipitation. Biochemistry 1997: 36: 5566–5577.

[49] Khanna S, Roy S, Bagchi D, Bagchi M, Sen CK. Upregulation of oxidant-induced VEGF expression in cultured keratinocytes by a grape seed proanthocyanidin extract. Free Radical Biology and Medicine 2001: 31(1): 38–42.

[50] Isaac O. Pharmacological investigations with compounds of chamomile, I. (-)-alpha-bisabolol and bisabolol oxides. Planta Medica 1979: 35: 118–124.

[51] Villegas LF, Marcalo A, Martin J, Fernaández ID, Maldonado H, Vaisberg AJ, Hammond GG. (+)-epi-Bisbolol Is the wound-healing principle of *Peperomia galioides*: investigation of the *in vivo* wound-healing activity of related terpenoids. Journal of Natural Products 2001: 64(10): 1357–1359.

[52] Shukla A, Rasik AM, Jain GK, Shankar R, Kulshrestha DK, Dhawan BN. In vitro and in vivo wound healing activity of asiaticoside isolated from *Centella asiatica*. Journal of Ethnopharmacology 1999: 65(1): 1–11.

[53] Singh SDJ, Krishna V, Mankani KL, Manjunata BK, Vidiya SM, Manohara YN. Wound healing activity of the leaf extracts and deoxyelephantopin isolated from *Elephantopus scaber* Linn. Indian Journal of Pharmacology 2005: 37(4): 238–242.

[54] Wicke C, Halliday B, Allen D, Roche NS, Scheuenstuh H, Spencer MM, Roberts AB, Hunt TK. Effects of steroids and retinoids on wound healing. Archives of Surgery 2000: 135(11): 1265–1270.

[55] Shim KM, Choi SH, Jeong MJ, Kang SS. Effects of aucubin on the healing of oral wounds. In Vivo 2007: 21(6): 1037–1041.

[56] Porras-Reyes BH, Lewis WH, Roman J, Simchowitz L, Mustoe TA. Enhancement of wound healing by the alkaloid taspine defining mechanism of action. Proceedings of the Society for Experimental Biology and Medicine 1993: 203(1): 18–25.

[57] Nesterova YV, Povetieva TN, Suslov NI, Zhdanov VV, Hrichkova TY, Udut EV, Chaykovskiy AS, Gaydamovich NN, Andreeva TI, Dygai AM. Regeneratory characteristics of complex extract and isolated diterpene alkaloids of *Aconitum baikalense*. Bulletin of Experimental Biology and Medicine 2012: 152(4): 439–443.

[58] Gowdru HB, Rajashekarappa S, Krishna V, Manjunatha HC. Molecular docking and evaluation of wound healing activity of stigmastatone isolated from bark of *Celastrus paniculatus* Willd. Journal of Biochemical Technology 2012: 3(5): S134–S137.

[59] Femenia A, Sanchez ES, Simal S, Rossello C. Compositional features of polysaccharides from *Aloe vera* (*Aloe barbadensis* Miller) plant tissues. Carbohydrate Polymers 1999: 39(2): 109–117. doi: 10.1016/S0144-8617(98)00163-5

[60] Djeraba A, Quere P. *In vivo* macrophage activation in chickens with Acemannan, a complex carbohydrate extracted from *Aloe vera*. International Journal of Immunopharmacology 2000: 22(5): 365–372. doi: 10.1016/S0192-0561(99)00091-0

[61] Castleman M. The Healing Herbs, Rodale Press, Emmaus, 1991: pp. 42–44.

[62] Syed TA, Afzal M, Ashfaq AS. Management of genital herpe in men with 0.5% *Aloe vera* extracts in a hydrophilic cream: a placebo-controlled double-blind study. Journal of Dermatological Treatment 1997: 8(2): 99–102. doi: 10.3109/09546639709160279

[63] Maheshwari RK, Singh AK, Gaddipati J, Srimal RC. Multiple biological activities of curcumin: a short review. Life Sciences 2006: 78(18): 2081–2087.

[64] Thangapazham RL, Sharma A, Maheshwari RK. Beneficial role of curcumin in skin diseases. Advances in Experimental and Medical Biology 2007: 595: 343–357.

[65] Panchatcharam M, Miriyala S, Gayathri VS, Suguna L. Curcumin improves wound healing by modulating collagen and decreasing reactive oxygen species. Molecular and Cellular Biochemistry 2006: 290(1–2): 87–96.

[66] Rao AB, Prasad E, Deepthi SS, Haritha V, Ramakrishna S, Madhusudan K, Surekha MV, Rao YSRV. Wound healing: a new perspective on glucosylated tetrahydrocurcumin. Drug Design Development and Therapy 2015: 9: 3579–3588.

Chapter 3

In Search of Wound Healing Drugs: A Journey Through Ayurveda

Tuhin K. Biswas, Saheli Banerjee, Nandini Poyra,
Srikanta Pandit, Utpalendu Jana,
Shrabana Chakrabarti and Tapan Seal

Additional information is available at the end of the chapter

http://dx.doi.org/10.5772/65520

Abstract

Description of wound healing is a recent concern of modern surgery and medical therapeutics, but first evidences are available in ancient Indian system of medicine, namely Ayurveda in the name of *Vrana* (wounds) and *Vranaropaka* (wound healing drugs). It has been reported that in different classical Ayurvedic texts, about 164 medicinal plants, 24 metals and minerals and 18 animal products are described for their wound healing activity. The mechanism of the healing process and the selection of drugs from natural resources are very specific in Ayurveda, and some of these have been scientifically screened. Besides a single component of drug, many classical formulations either in the form of polyherbal or herbo-minerals have been cited in Ayurveda from time to time since pre-vedic era to recent modern time. Many traditional folkloric preparations of India were also later on incorporated in Ayurveda utilizing sources of some pockets of Ayurveda in different parts of the country. Chronological development of these drugs on the basis of physical, molecular and clinical parameters is elaborated vividly with some examples of experimentation like *Curcuma longa, Pterocarpus santalinus, Cynodon dactylon* and a composed formulation named *Kshantak Malam*.

Keywords: wound healing, Ayurveda, *Vranaropaka*, medicinal plants, metals and minerals

1. Introduction

The development of drugs for wound management is a concern of long history in medical science, and probably it was first described in Indian system of medicine, *Ayurveda*. Healing of wound is a natural phenomenon, but the natural way of healing may lack quality, promptness and aesthetics [1]. Biology of wound healing involves a phases like homeostasis and fibrin deposition, inflammation, wound debridement, neoangiognesis, fibroblast proliferation, scar modulation, wound contraction and epithelisation [2]. In recent studies, many drugs and/or agents are reported for management of wounds. Silver is being used since a long back for the management of wounds specially for its antibacterial property [3]. The highly reactive charged silver ion (Ag^+) reacts by binding to negatively charged particles such as proteins, DNA, RNA and chloride ions. While this is responsible for its antimicrobial properties, it also complicates delivery as the silver ions are readily bound to proteins and chloride in the wound bed fluid [4]. Acute conditions of wounds are now being treated by non-pharmacological procedures like negative pressure wound device (NPWD) or vacuum assisted closure (VAC) [5] and hydrogel [6]. Several synthetic growth factors like vascular endothelial growth factor (VEGF), platelet derived growth factor (PDGF), epidermal growth factor (EGF), transforming growth factor-β (TGF-β), insulin-like growth factor-I (IGF-I), etc. are reported to have healing properties in specific types of wounds on pre-clinical models [7]. The specific role of EGF is documented as a topical application in cutaneous wounds [8]. These agents performed such activities by stimulating fibroblast proliferation and keratinocytes via transmembrane glycoproteins [9]. The use of NPWD or VAC is limited to stable wounds while hydrogel is applicable in moist wounds. The basic types of fibroblast growth factor (bFGF) is a variety, which stimulates the healing process and inhibits scar formation but may have several side effects like irritation, pain, erythema, pruritis, etc. [10]. However, cost of growth factors therapy in wound healing may not be accessible to common people, and some of the growth factors like recombinant human growth hormone (rhGH) and recombinant human insulin like growth factor-I (rhIGF-I) are reported to have serious side effects like fluid retention, gynecomastia or orthostatic hypotension, specially in elderly patients [11].

In Ayurveda, the Indian system of medicine, elaborative description about the treatment of wounds is mentioned, particularly in the text, *Sushruta Samhita* (ca. 1000 BC), in the name of '*Vrana*' or wounds [12]. In describing the pathogenesis of wound or *Vrana*, three stages are mentioned in Sushruta Samhita as unsuppurtaed (*Ama* stage) wound, early suppurated (*Pachyamana* stage) wound and fully suppurated (*Pakva* stage) wound. Specific symptoms are mentioned for different stages of wounds in this text. A series of 60 steps of treatment for wounds (*Sasti Vrana Upakrama*) is mentioned in Ayurveda, which starts with dissolution of inflammation and ends with correction of deformities in the wound area. Out of these series of 60 steps of treatment, seven steps are most important and one of which is use of plants, minerals and animal products as *Vranaropaka Dravyas* (wound healing agents). This divergence of Ayurvedic drugs definitely excel those of modern remedies for the wounds, but a very few of those have been screened in a scientific way to prove their efficacy. In different classical Ayurvedic texts, about 164 medicinal plants, 24 metals and minerals and 18 animal products are described for their wound healing activity under the term '*Vranaropaka*' [13]. Some of these

http://dx.doi.org/10.5772/65520

agents are already reported for potentiality in management of wounds which are being described in present review.

2. Review of wound healing drugs in Ayurveda

2.1. Plant drugs

Description of wound healing drugs is found in different Ayurvedic texts of different era. It has been observed that there were development in compositions and selection of more specific drugs of natural resources towards specific therapeutic activity, particularly wound healing *per se*, according to chronological changes of different periods. Systemic development of Ayurvedic therapies, particularly with plant origin, is found during sixth century BC to seventh century AD when classical texts like *Charaka Samhita, Sushruta Samhita* and *Astanga Hridaya* were written. The text *Sushruta Samhita* particularly describes the surgical aspects of therapeutics including wound healing through 120 chapters in 5 cantos. However, treatment for wounds in these texts was detailed in the form of multi-ingredient compositions (polyherbal or herbo-mineral). Later on during the period between tenth and sixteenth centuries AD, use of single medicinal plants was emphasized for specific therapeutic purpose like wound healing. The classical text like *Bhavaprakash Nighantu* was written during this period [14]. All these changes from time to time were incorporated owing to the pieces of evidence acquired from the therapeutic experiences by Ayurvedic physicians. In search of this development on wound healing drugs of Ayurvedic origin, a total number of 164 medicinal plants are found to be cited in various classical texts [15]. These medicinal plants are categorized under 73 families with highest number of inclusion under Leguminosae having 20 medicinal plants followed by Compositeae with eight medicinal plants (**Table 1**). Besides families of inclusion, it is also important to know that which part of the plant is responsible for the wound healing property. There is very much specificity of plant parts used for wound healing activity according to variations in plants as described in Ayurveda. It is reported that different plant parts like leaves, root, seed, stem (whole stem, heart wood and stem bark), flowers, fruits (pulp and whole plant), gum, rhizome, latex, filament and whole plants are used for the said purpose owing to specificity of their chemical compositions [15]. Gum and latex may be considered as secondary metabolites of the plants. It has been observed that among 164 medicinal plants described for wound healing, mostly roots (45) are used for therapeutic purpose (**Table 1**). Pieces of scientific evidence of some of these species are being described here for their wound healing properties.

2.1.1. Curcuma longa

The rhizome of *Curcuma longa* L. (family Zingiberaceae), which is commonly known as turmeric, has been widely used for centuries in traditional medicines for several diseases, with the biological actions like antioxidant, anticarcinogenic, anti-inflammatory, antimutagenic, antimicrobial and hypocholesteraemic activities [16]. Most of these biological activities are due to presence of its main bioactive component curcumin (**Figure 1**). The wound healing property of the plant has been particularly described in the text 'Bhavaprakash Nighantu' [17].

Sl	Family	Total no. of plants cited	Parts of plants used with number distribution										
			Leaves	Stem	Flower	Fruit	Root	Seed	Gum	Rhizome	Latex	Filament	Whole plant
	Acanthaceae	01	01	–	–	–	–	–	–	–	–	–	–
	Algae	01	–	–	–	–	–	–	–	–	–	01	–
	Amaranthaceae	02	–	–	–	–	–	–	–	–	–	–	02
	Anacardaceae	03	01	01	–	–	01	–	–	–	–	–	–
	Anonaceae	01	01	–	–	–	–	–	–	–	–	–	–
	Apocyanaceae	04	01	01	–	–	02	–	–	–	–	–	–
	Araceae	01	–	–	–	–	–	–	–	01	–	–	–
	Aristolochiaceae	01	–	–	–	–	–	–	–	–	–	–	01
	Asclepidiaceae	04	01	–	–	–	02	–	–	–	01	–	–
10	Berberidaceae	01	–	01	–	–	–	–	–	–	–	–	–
11	Bombacaceae	01	–	01	–	–	–	–	–	–	–	–	–
12	Boraginaceae	01	01	–	–	–	–	–	–	–	–	–	–
13	Capparidaceae	02	–	–	–	–	02	–	–	–	–	–	–
14	Celestraceae	01	–	–	–	–	–	01	–	–	–	–	–
15	Combretaceae	03	–	01	–	02	–	–	–	–	–	–	–
16	Compositeae	08	02	01	01	–	03	01	–	–	–	–	–
17	Convolvulaceae	02	–	–	–	-	02	–	–	–	–	–	–
18	Cucurbitaceae	05	02	–	–	–	02	01	–	–	–	–	–
19	Cyperaceae	01	–	–	–	–	01	–	–	–	–	–	–
20	Dipterocarpaceae	02	–	–	–	–	–	–	01	–	01	–	–
21	Euphorbiaceae	05	01	–	–	01	–	01	–	–	01	–	01
22	Gentinaceae	01	–	01	–	–	–	–	–	–	–	–	–
23	Gramineae	06	–	–	–	–	03	02	–	–	–	–	01
24	Gutaceae	01	–	–	–	–	–	–	–	–	–	–	01
25	Gutiferae	01	–	–	01	–	–	–	–	–	–	–	–
26	Hydrophyllaceae	01	–	–	–	–	01	–	–	–	–	–	–
27	Irideae	02	–	01	01	–	–	–	–	–	–	–	–
28	Lauraceae	01	–	01	–	–	–	–	–	–	–	–	–
29	Labiateae	01	–	–	–	–	–	–	–	–	–	–	01
30	Leguminosae	20	02	03	–	–	03	09	01	–	–	–	02
31	Liliaceae	02	–	–	–	–	02	–	–	–	–	–	–
32	Loranthaceae	01	–	–	–	–	–	–	–	–	–	–	01
33	Lytheraceae	01	–	–	01	–	–	–	–	–	–	–	–
34	Malvaceae	03	–	–	–	01	02	–	–	–	–	–	–
35	Meliaceae	01	–	–	–	–	01	–	–	–	–	–	–
36	Menispermaceae	02	–	01	–	–	01	–	–	–	–	–	–

Sl	Family	Total no. of plants cited	Parts of plants used with number distribution										
			Leaves	Stem	Flower	Fruit	Root	Seed	Gum	Rhizome	Latex	Filament	Whole plant
37	Mimosoiodeae	02	–	01	–	–	–	–	–	–	–	–	01
38	Moraceae	05	01	03	–	01	–	–	–	–	–	–	–
39	Moringaceae	01	–	–	–	–	01	–	–	–	–	–	–
40	Musaceae	01	–	01	–	–	–	–	–	–	–	–	–
41	Myricaceae	01	–	01	–	–	–	–	–	–	–	–	–
42	Myrsinaceae	01	–	–	–	01	–	–	–	–	–	–	–
43	Myrtaceae	01	–	01	–	–	–	–	–	–	–	–	–
44	Mertyneaceae	01	–	–	–	01	–	–	–	–	–	–	–
45	Nyctaginaceae	01	–	–	–	–	–	–	–	–	–	–	01
46	Nymphaeceae	04	–	01	–	–	03	–	–	–	–	–	–
47	Oleaceae	03	01	–	01	01	–	–	–	–	–	–	–
48	Orchidaceae	01	–	–	–	–	01	–	–	–	–	–	–
49	Papavaraceae	01	–	–	–	–	–	01	–	–	–	–	–
50	Papilionaceae	01	–	01	–	–	–	–	–	–	–	–	–
51	Pedaliaceae	01	–	–	–	–	–	01	–	–	–	–	–
52	Pinaceae	02	01	–	–	–	–	01	–	–	–	–	–
53	Piperaceae	04	–	–	–	03	01	–	–	–	–	–	–
54	Plumbaginaceae	01	–	–	–	–	01	–	–	–	–	–	–
55	Polypoidiaceae	01	01	–	–	–	–	–	–	–	–	–	–
56	Rannunculaceae	01	–	–	–	–	–	–	–	–	–	–	01
57	Rosaceae	03	–	01	–	–	01	01	–	–	–	–	–
58	Rubiaceae	04	–	02	–	–	01	–	–	–	–	–	01
59	Rutaceae	04	02	–	–	01	01	–	–	–	–	–	–
60	Salicaceae	01	–	01	–	–	–	–	–	–	–	–	–
61	Santalanaceae	01	–	01	–	–	–	–	–	–	–	–	–
62	Sapotaceae	02	–	01	–	–	–	–	–	–	–	–	–
63	Scrophulariaceae	01	–	–	–	–	–	–	–	01	–	–	–
64	Simaronbaceae	01	–	01	–	–	–	–	–	–	–	–	–
65	Solanaceae	02	01	–	–	–	01	–	–	–	–	–	–
66	Symplocaceae	01	–	01	–	–	–	–	–	–	–	–	–
67	Thymelaceae	01	–	–	–	–	–	–	01	–	–	–	–
68	Tiliaceae	01	–	01	–	–	–	–	–	–	–	–	–
69	Umbeliferae	02	–	–	–	01	01	–	–	–	–	–	–
70	Valerianaceae	01	–	–	–	–	01	–	–	–	–	–	–
71	Verbenaceae	04	02	–	–	01	01	–	–	–	–	–	–
72	Zingiberaceae	06	–	–	–	–	01	02	–	03	–	–	–
73	Zygophyllaceae	01	–	–	–	01	–	–	–	–	–	–	–
Total	164	22	31	05	13	45	21	04	05	03	01	14	

Table 1. Categorisation of medicinal plants reported in classical Ayurvedic texts for wound healing activity.

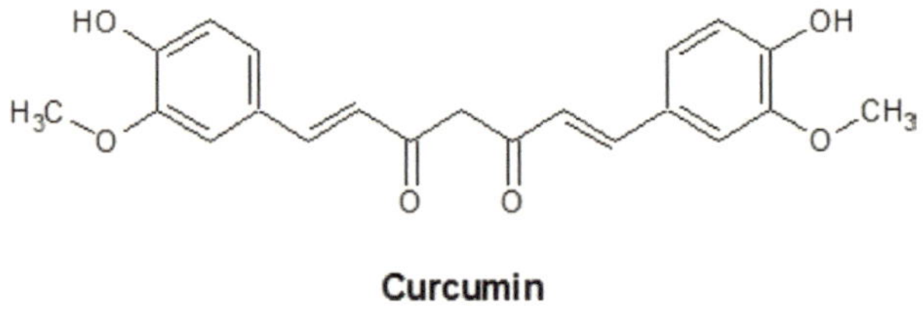

Figure 1. Chemical structure of curcumin.

Pre-clinical investigation of this plant was performed for wound healing activity in a rabbit model in comparison with honey. Significant ($p < 0.01$) improvement of the tensile strength and wound contraction (mm^2) was observed with *C. longa* within a period of 14 days to heal a rectangular full thickness wound measuring $10 \times 4\ cm^2$ area. The result was further evaluated on the basis of the histopathological parameters revealing well-organized remodelling of collagen, reticulin and elastin fibres as well as appearance of epithelialisation and neovascularisation [18]. It has been postulated that the cross linking of collagen for the purpose of wound healing with curcumin is due to its antioxidant properties [19].

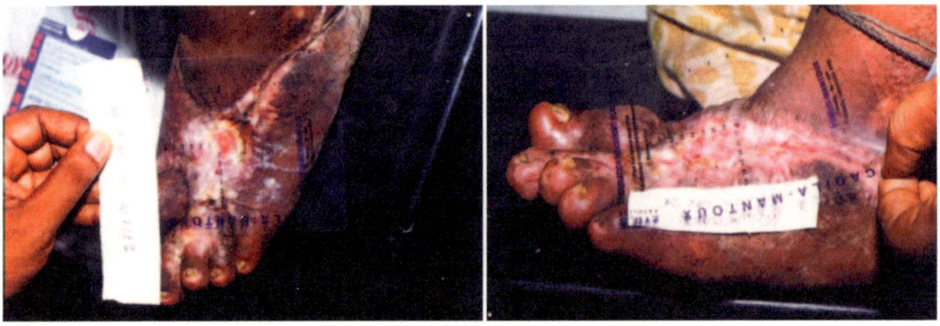

a **b**

Figure 2. Patient of lower extremity wound before (a) and after (b) 15 days treatment with 15% *P. santalinus ointment.*

2.1.2. *Pterocarpus santalinus*

The heartwood of the plant *Pterocarpus santalinus* L. (family Papilionaceae), commonly known in the name of red sandal wood, is described in Ayurveda for wound healing property [20]. A detailed wound healing study in the pharmacological model on Charles Foster strain rats was performed on 8 mm full thickness punch, burn and streptozotocin-induced wound models. Significant ($p < 0.001$) results were observed on the basis of the wound contraction size, tensile strength, tissue DNA, RNA, protein and collagen (hydroxyproline as a marker) synthesis, tissue remodelling as observed by histological studies on collagenesis, angiogenesis and epithelialisation [21]. The results were finally quantified by PAGE study with estimation of protein synthesis in which it was found that proteins with different molecular weight on the variations in different days were synthesised indicating its potentiality in triggering the cell signalling system for successful healing of the wounds. A pilot clinical study on selected six patients of lower extremity wounds was evaluated with 15% paste of the drug under ointment base and significant ($p < 0.01$) improvement was observed (**Figure 2**) on the basis of the granulation and epithelialisation [22]. The drug has been patented officially and now being marketed either as single ingredient or in combined form for the purpose of wound healing.

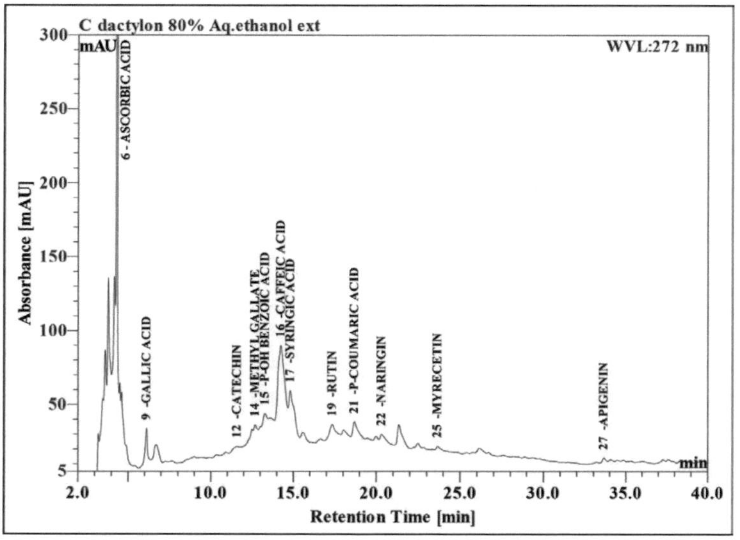

Figure 3. HPLC chromatogram of 80% aq. ethanol extract of *C. dactylon*.

2.1.3. Cynodon dactylon

Cynodon dactylon (Linn.) Pers (Family Gramineae) is a medicinal plant categorized in Ayurveda for its wound healing activity. In *Charaka Samhita*, one of the oldest classical text of Ayurveda, the plant is described in different names for different activities such as '*Sita*' and '*Lata*' for its role to improve body complexion, '*Satavirya*' and '*Sahasravirya*' for its fertility promoting activity, etc. and '*Durva*' for use as fresh juice in the treatment of wounds (*Vrana*) in particular [23]. A detailed chemical, pharmacological and clinical study of 80% aqueous ethanol extract of the plant was performed by the authors for wound healing activity. Chemical study with HPLC revealed that the extract of the plant was found to contain total phenol (23.98 ± 0.16 mg/g GAE), flavonoid (5.79 ± 0.14 mg/g rutin equivalent) and flavonol (14.84 ± 0.17 mg/g quercetin equivalent) (**Figure 3**). The plant also showed antiradical activity by scavenging DPPH (IC_{50} 2.29 ± 0.13 mg/g) and ABTS radical (IC_{50} 0.40 ± 0.001 mg/g). The HPLC analysis of the crude ethanol extract of the plant under investigation showed the presence of ascorbic acid (7.66 ± 0.05 mg/g), phenolic acids namely gallic acid (0.44 ± 0.01 mg/g), *p*-hydroxy benzoic acid (0.06 ± 0.009 mg/g), caffeic acid (2.20 ± 0.01 mg/g), syringic acid (2.78 ± 0.02 mg/g), *p*-coumaric acid (0.44 ± 0.006 mg/g), flavonoids like rutin (0.88 ± 0.01 mg/g), naringin (0.14 ± 0.003 mg/g), myricetin (0.08 ± 0.002 mg/g), apigenin (0.05 ± 0.0009 mg/g) and catechin (0.58 ± 0.006 mg/g) (**Tables 2** and **3**). The phenolic acids and flavonoids present in the plant can react with the reactive oxygen species and act as free radical scavengers leading to healing of wounds [24]. Detailed experimental study on an 8 mm full thickness punch wound in CF rats showed that the 5% ointment prepared with aqueous ethanol extract of the plant could significantly be able to contract the wounds within a very short period of 10 days and could generate tissue protein, DNA, RNA, protein and hydroxyproline, which were significantly ($p < 0.05$–0.01) better than standard comparator framycetin topical antibiotic ointment or vehicle control petroleum jelly (**Table 4**). The pharmacological study thus conspicuously mimics the chemical analysis of the plant. The drug, thereafter, clinically evaluated by selecting 12 patients of non-healing wounds dividing into two groups comprising equal number (6) of patients treating with 5% ointment prepared with aqueous ethanol extract of the plant and standard comparator framycetin topical antibiotic ointment continuously applied for 21 days. Physical examination on the basis of wound contraction (mm^2) and appearance of granulation and epithelialisation showed significant improvement ($p < 0.05$) in *C. dactylon* treated group than the comparator (**Table 5**).

Name of the plant	Total phenolic content mg/g dry extract (GAE equivalent)	Total flavonoid content mg/g dry extract (rutin equivalent)	Total flavonol content mg/g dry extract (quercetin equivalent)	Reducing power mg/g dry extract (AAE equivalent)	DPPH radical scavenging activity IC_{50} mg/g dry extract	ABTS radical scavenging activity IC_{50} mg/g dry extract
C. dactylon	23.9 ± 0.16	5.79 ± 0.14	14.84 ± 0.17	12.96 ± 0.68	2.29 ± 0.13	0.40 ± 0.001

Each value in the table was obtained by calculating the average of three experiments and data presented as mean ± SEM.

Table 2. Total phenolic, flavonoid, flavonol content, reducing power and radical scavenging activities of 80% aq. ethanol extract of *C. dactylon*.

Ascorbic acid/phenolic acids/flavonoids in *C. dactylon*	Amount in mg/g dry extract (mean ± SD)
Ascorbic acid	7.66 ± 0.05
Gallic acid	0.44 ± 0.01
Catechin	0.58 ± 0.006
Methyl gallate	0.12 ± 0.01
p-Hydroxy benzoic acid	0.06 ± 0.009
Caffeic acid	2.20 ± 0.01
Syringic acid	2.78 ± 0.02
Rutin	0.88 ± 0.01
p-Coumaric acid	0.44 ± 0.006
Naringin	0.14 ± 0.003
Myricetin	0.08 ± 0.002
Apigenin	0.05 ± 0.0009

Table 3. Quantification of ascorbic acids, phenolic acids and flavonoids in the 80% aq. ethanol extract of *C. dactylon*.

http://dx.doi.org/10.5772/65520

Physical and biochemical parameters	*C. dactylon* (n = 6)	Framycetin (n = 6)	Petroleum jelly (vehicle) (n = 6)
Wound contraction (mm^2)	2.04 ± 0.48*	2.64 ± 0.70	3.33 ± 0.31
Healing period (days)	10.00 ± 0.97*	12.00 ± 0.63*	15.83 ± 0.93
Tensile strength (g)	421.50 ± 32.84*	410.41 ± 34.57	301.12 ± 24.08
DNA (mg/g)	2.02 ± 0.05*	2.49 ± 0.02*	1.11 ± 0.06
RNA (mg/g)	1.92 ± 0.03*	2.13 ± 0.02*	1.01 ± 0.02
Protein (mg/g)	22.73 ± 0.06**	25.16 ± 0.10**	12.30 ± 0.15
Hydroxyproline (mg/g)	4.69 ± 0.06**	3.72 ± 0.07**	1.99 ± 0.05

Results are expressed in mean ± SEM.
$^*p < 0.05$.
$^{**}p < 0.01$.

Table 4. Physical and biochemical assessment of 5% *C. dactylon* ointment with respect to vehicle control and framycetin in punch wound model in rat.

Parameters	Time interval (n = 6)	*C. dactylon* (n = 6)	Framycetin (n = 6)
Wound area (mm^2)	0 day	25.58	15.00
	21 day	0.37	0
	d ± SE	25.06 ± 5.25*	15.00 ± 2.83*
Granulation/epithelialisation	0 day	1.11	1.00
	21 day	4.96	1.33
	d ± SE	3.86 ± 0.08*	0.33 ± 0.23

Results are expressed in mean differences (d) ± SE.
$^*p < 0.05$.

Table 5. Physical evaluation of 5% *C. dactylon* ointment in comparison with framycetin treated group in patients of chronic non-healing wounds.

2.1.4. Polyherbal formulation

Most of the drugs in Ayurveda are used in the polyherbal form for different diseases. These formulations were standardized in the composition and preparation technique according to the clinical experiences obtained from time to time as well as experiences gained from one group of Ayurvedic School to other. A classic example is also applied in designing wound healing drugs of polyherbal composition developed by Bengal school of Ayurveda. The unique preparation is commonly known in the local name of '*Kshatantak Malam*' (wound healing ointment), prepared with leaves of *Achyranthesaspera* L. (Amaranthaceae), onion juice (*Allium cepa* L., Lilliaceae) and leaves of *Cannabis sativa* L (Cannabaceae) under the base of butter. The whole preparation is placed in a decanted tender coconut and covered well with clothes and mud. The preparation when dried is put in a pit and fired by natural way with cow dung cakes (**Figure 4a–d**). The ointment thus obtained was chemically screened by gas liquid chromatography (GLC), which showed presence of palmitic acid, oleic acid and polyunsaturated fatty acids. It was rendered for detailed pharmacological screening through the standard protocol after initial acute and chronic toxicity studies in the mice model, revealing safe in use. Pharmacologically the drug showed very significant ($p < 0.05$) wound healing activity when screened on the basis of the physical parameters like wound contraction size, wound index, healing period, tensile strength; biochemical marker evaluation like tissue DNA, RNA, protein, hydroyproline and PAGE study and histological findings [25]. A multidimensional *modus operandi* is proposed for wound healing activity of this formulation. The formulation is composed with *Acyranthes aspera, Allium cepa* and *Cannabis sativa. A. aspera* is earlier reported for potent activity in diabetic, burn and immune compromised wounds. *A. cepa* is reported to be active against several micro-organisms like *Streptococcus aureus, Bacilus subtilis* and *Pseudomonas aeruginosa* supporting its anti-bacterial. Butter is used as a good homogenous substance. *C. sativa*, on the other hand, has capability to repair tissues due to its anti-inflammatory property [25].

2.2. Metals and minerals

Metals and minerals are used in Ayurveda to combat several diseases. However, there is description of the technical procedure for purification of these components before therapeutic use. *Jasada bhasma*, an Ayurvedic preparation of zinc, is used for the treatment of wounds. In a pre-clinical study, 10 and 20% ointment of *Jasad Bhasma* was screened both in incised and excised wounds, which showed increased wound contraction and tensile strength, decreased period of re-epithelization and scar area along with proliferative activity on fibroblasts. It is proposed that the functional role of zinc in repair systems is provided by demonstration of zinc metalloenzymes like alkaline phosphatase, RNA and DNA polymerases and metalloproteinases [26].

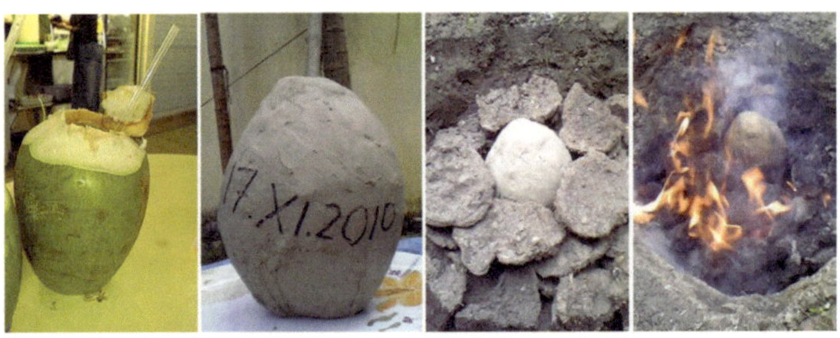

a b c d

Figure 4. Steps of preparation of *Kshantak Malam* initiated with decanted tender coconut (a), putting of drug preparation covering with clothes and mud (b), placing on pit with cow dung cakes (c) and firing till the end of reaction (d).

2.3. Animal products

Besides, medicinal plants and metallic drugs, animal products also play an important role in treatment of wounds in Ayurveda. The most important animal products that exhibit wound healing activity is honey. Several studies are reported for wound healing potential of honey. Honey performed the healing activity due to its anti-oxidant, anti-inflammatory, wound debridement, leukocytic stimulation, cytokine and growth factor releasing as well as osmotic activities probably due to presence of natural phenolic compounds [27].

3. Conclusion

Healing of wounds engrosses a diverse mechanism in the process of cell repair involving multiple biological factors. Ideal healing is demarcated with successful closure of wounds in minimum days without any adverse effect. Ayurveda is one of the best ethnological sources to search natural sources for wound healing property. Many drugs are described in different texts for wound healing property, but only few of them have been scientifically screened which are described in the recent review. The information provided in favour of *C. dactylon,* is purely unpublished and may have potentiality in future. Other drugs of Ayurvedic origin either plants, metals or animal origin already exist in clinical practice for wound healing purpose.

Acknowledgements

Authors are thankful to Professor Biswapati Mukherjee, former Director, S. N. Pradhan Centre for Neuroscience, University of Calcutta for encouragement. Authors are also thankful to the Indian Council of Medical Research for financial support to conduct research on *Kshanatak Malam.*

Author details

Tuhin K. Biswas[1*], Saheli Banerjee[1], Nandini Poyra[1], Srikanta Pandit[1], Utpalendu Jana[1], Shrabana Chakrabarti[1] and Tapan Seal[2]

*Address all correspondence to: biswastuhin@rediffmail.com

1 Research Unit, J. B. Roy State Ayurvedic Medical College and Hospital, Kolkata, India

2 Department of Plant Chemistry, Botanical Survey of India, Howrah, India

References

[1] Ramesh KV, Wound repair: drug research and therapeutics, Ann. Update in Clin. Pharmacol., Ind. Pharmacol. Soc., 1993, 1: 13–8.

[2] Ganguli AC, Wound healing. In: Wound Healing and Wound Care, Roussel India, Ltd., Bombay, India, 1994, pp. 15–19.

[3] Warriner R and Burrell R, Infection and the chronic wound: a focus on silver, Adv skin Wound Care, 2005, 18: 2–12.

[4] Mooney EK, Lippitt C, and Friedman J, Silver dressings [safety and efficacy reports], Plast Reconstr Surg, 2006, 117 (2): 666–669.

[5] Argenta LC, Morykwas MJ, Marks MW, DeFranzo AJ, Molnar JA, and David LR, Vacuum-assisted closure: state of clinic art, Plast Reconstr Surg, 2006, 117 (7): 127S–142S.

[6] Morin RJ and Tomaselli NL, Interactive dressings and topical agents, Clin Plast Surg, 2007, 34(4): 643–658.

[7] Kiritsy CP, and Lynch SE, Role of growth factors in cutaneous wound healing: a review, Crit Rev Oral Biol Med, 1993, 4(5): 729–760.

[8] Brown GL, Nanney LB, Griffen J, Cramer AB, Yancey JM, Curtsinger LJ, Holtzin L, Schultz GS, Jurkiewicz MJ, and Lynch JB, Enhancement of wound healing by topical treatment with epidermal growth factor, New Engl J Med, 1989, 321: 76–79.

[9] Bennett SAL and Birnboim HC, Receptor-mediated and protein kinase-dependent growth enhancement of primary human fibroblasts by platelet activating factor, Mol Carcinog, 1997, 20 (4): 366–375.

[10] Okabe K, Hayashi R, Aramaki-Hattori,Yoshiaki Sakamoto N, and Kishi K, Wound treatment using growth factors, Modern Plastic Surg, 2013, 3: 108–112

[11] Sullivan DH, Carter WJ, Warr WR, and Williams LH, Side effects resulting from the use of growth hormone and insulin like growth factor-I as combined therapy to frail elderly patients, J Gerontol Med Sci, 1998, 53A (3): M183–M187.

[12] Dash B and Kashyap L, Diagnosis and treatment of diseases in Ayurveda, Concept Publishing Co., New Delhi, 1980, Vol. 4. pp. 500–598.

[13] Biswas TK and Mukherjee B, Plant medicine of Indian origin for wound healing activity: a review, Int J Lower Extrem Wounds, 2003, 2 (1): 25–39.

[14] Narayanaswamy V, Origin and development of Ayurveda (a brief history), Ancient Sci Life, 1981, 1 (1): 1–7.

[15] Biswas TK and Mukherjee B, Plant medicine of Indian origin for wound healing activity: a review, Int J Lower Extrem Wounds, 2003, 2 (1): 25–39.

[16] Gritsanapan W and Pothitirat, Traditional herbs for health care – turmeric: a case history. In: Evaluation of Herbal Medicianl Products, Pharmaceutical Press, London, 2009, pp. 322–339.

[17] Bhavamishra, Bhavaprakasha, PurvaKhanda and MadhyamKhanda, HarityakadiVarga and Vranadhikara, Hindi Commentary by Bramha Shankar Mishra, 8th Ed, Varanasi, UP, India, Chaukkhamba Sanskrit Bhavan, 2003, pp. 170–194, 258–270.

[18] Kundu S, Biswas TK, Das P, Kumar S, and De DK, Turmeric (*Curcuma longa*) rhizome paste and honey show similar wound healing potential: a preclinical study in rabbits, Int J Lower Extrem Wounds, 2005, 4(4): 205–213.

[19] Panchatcharama M, Miriyala S, Gayathri VS, and Suguna L, Curcumin improves wound healing by modulating collagen and decreasing reactive oxygen species, Mol Cell Biochem, 2006, 290: 87–96.

[20] Kirtikar KR and Basu BD, Indian Medicinal Plants, Vol. 1, Periodical Experts, India, 1981.

[21] Biswas TK, Maity LN, and Mukherjee B, Wound healing potential of *Pterocarpus santalinus* Linn.: a pharmacological evaluation, Int J Lower Extrem Wounds, 2004, 3(3): 143–150.

[22] Biswas TK, Maity LN, and Mukherjee B, The clinical evaluation of *Pterocarpus santalinus* Linn. ointment on lower extremity wounds: a preliminary report, Int J Lower Extrem Wounds, 2004, 3(4): 227–232.

[23] Sharma RK and Dash B (Eds.), Charaka Samhita, Sutrasthana, Vol. I and IV, Chapter IV and XXV, Chowkhamba Sanskrit Series Office, Varanasi, 2007, 88–101: 459–460.

[24] Kamath JV, Rana AC, and Chaudhary AR, Prohealing effect of *Cinnamomumzeylenicum* bark. Phytother Res, 2003, 17: 970–972.

[25] Gangopadhyay KS, Khan M, Pandit S, Chakrabarti S, Mondal TK, and Biswas TK, Pharmacological evaluation and chemical standardization of an Ayurvedic formulation for wound healing activity, Int J Lower Ext Wounds, 2014, 13 (1): 41–49.

[26] Shah DP, Sathaye S, and Korde A, Pharmacologicl evaluation of wound healing potential of *Jasad Bhasma* using Wistar rats: a mechanistic approach, *Pharmacologyonline*, 2009, 2: 1269–1277.

[27] Molan PC, The evidence and rationale for the use of honey as wound dressing, Wound Prac Res, 2011, 19(4): 204–220.

Chapter 4

Natural Compounds for Wound Healing

Mihaela Georgescu, Oana Marinas, Marcela Popa,
Teodora Stan, Veronica Lazar,
Serban Vifor Bertesteanu and
Mariana Carmen Chifiriuc

Additional information is available at the end of the chapter

http://dx.doi.org/10.5772/65652

Abstract

Many plants or plant-derived compounds with high levels of antioxidants and anti-inflammatory, immunomodulatory, and antimicrobial properties could be of great benefit for wound healing. Several studies have documented the use of plant extracts for the development of bioactive wound dressings. The purpose of this chapter is to give an update about the vegetal and bee products, which can be used as bioactive substances in wound dressings or in other formulations for wound healing. The adverse effects of plant and bee extracts, such as contact allergies, are also presented. In order to better exploit the huge reservoir of pharmacologically active plant-derived compounds and extracts, standardized methodology and clinical trials are necessary to give more concrete evidence supporting the use of traditional medicine in wound management.

Keywords: wound healing, essential oils, plant compounds, propolis, antimicrobial, immunomodulatory, antioxidant, wound dressings, dermatitis

1. Introduction

Wound healing is a complex and dynamic process which is not fully understood [1]. Leg ulcers are caused by circulatory problems and are characterized by the lack of skin substance, having a chronic evolution and delayed healing [2]. The causes of ulcers are (i) a prolonged or excessive inflammatory phase [3], (ii) persistent infections produced by microbial biofilms resistant to treatment, and (iii) failure of the epidermal or/and dermal cells to respond to the reparatory stimuli [4]. The characteristics of ulcers are an increased enzymatic activity of the matrix proteases, a low response to growth factors, and increased cell death [1].

Wounds and ulcers affect the patients' life quality with an annual cost of $25 treatment [5].

Medicinal plants have been used for thousands of years, worldwide, as traditional treatments for numerous diseases. For example, 65 herbs were used in the traditional Persian medicine, a holistic system of medicine, providing valuable information on natural remedies [6]. Almost 80 % of the population of developing countries, but also economy leaders as China and India, use traditional medicine for the treatment of a wide range of diseases [7, 8]. The naturally derived products from medicinal plants have proven to be an abundant source of biological active compounds, of which many have been used to start the development of new chemicals for the pharmaceutical industry.

There are approximately 500,000 species of plants in the world of which only 1 % have been phytochemically analyzed demonstrating a great potential for the discovery of new bioactive compounds [9]. Phytochemicals are nonnutritive substances present in plants, enhancing tissue remodeling when applied on wounds and acting as pro-angiogenic agents for wound healing [7]. From the 1184 new chemical entities introduced between 1981 and 2006, approximately half of them (48 %) were natural products, semisynthetic analogs of the natural products, or synthetic compounds based on the natural pharmacophores. Over 70 % of the therapeutic agents developed between 1981 and 2006 for bacterial and fungal infectious diseases have been derived from natural compounds [10, 11].

The therapeutic properties of vegetal extracts include the following effects, which are due either to some specific phytocompounds or to their synergic actions: anti-infectious, anticancer, antioxidant, immunomodulatory, actions on the central nervous system and on the cardiovascular system, and hemotropic activity.

Regarding the infectious diseases, the increased resistance of known pathogens to the currently used therapeutic agents, such as antibiotics and antiviral agents, has led to regaining the interest for the discovery of novel natural compounds with anti-infectious activity. The increasing appreciation of the different biological effects of the natural compounds has led to a reevaluation of the possible roles that these compounds play in plants, especially in the context of ecological interactions [12].

Besides the principal metabolites which assure the plant's viability, the plants produce many organic compounds, known as secondary metabolites, which do not participate directly to the growth and development of the plants. These are distributed differently in the taxonomic groups of the plants regnum. Many of their functions are not known, although they are remarkable through the complexity of their chemical structures and the biosynthesis pathways.

Many of these compounds are recognized, presently, as being involved in the plant's defense, having an insecticide, antimicrobial, and repellent effect; in reproduction, they have a role of attractant for pollinators and act as allelopathic agents. These ecological functions affect the survival of the plants and, apparently, the secondary metabolites of plants' act, mainly, on other species, being known the fact that invasive plants produce compounds that stop the development of autochthonous species in the clonal area [12].

This chapter is a synthesis of original results published in the PhD works of the chapter coauthors and also of research articles available from PubMed, using the following key words:

"wound healing" in association with one of the following "alternative methods" for "plant-derived compounds," "essential oils," "propolis," "*Calendula officinalis*," "aloe vera," "curcumin," "side effects," and "wound management."

2. Biological activities of plant compounds useful in the wound-healing process

2.1. Volatile oils

The volatile oils are products of the secondary vegetal metabolism, secreted by specialized cells, organized in different organs, and deposited in vacuoles, bags and secretory channels, or in the glandular hairs under the form of volatile liquids, oily, with nice, flavored scent. They are mixtures of different chemical compounds with different therapeutic properties [13]. Out of the 100,000 secondary known metabolites, the essential oils represent over 3000, of which approximately 300 have a commercial interest and are used in the food, cosmetic, and pharmaceutical industries [14].

2.1.1. The mechanisms of the antimicrobial action of the volatile oils

Over time, several mechanisms of action of the volatile oils on microbial cells have been proposed. The volatile oils can affect the cell wall and the cytoplasmatic compounds. Their hydrophobic character is, apparently, responsible for the perturbation of the bacterial structures. The mechanisms of action of the volatile oils include the degradation of the cell wall; the deterioration of the cytoplasmatic membrane; the cytoplasmatic coagulation; the deterioration of the membrane's proteins; and the increase of the permeability, which leads to the loss of the cellular content, reducing the proton force; and the intracellular ATP by decreasing the ATP synthesis [15].

The effect on the cellular membrane fatty acid profile: the adaptation of the microbial cells to a concentration lower than the minimal inhibitory concentration has been shown to lead to an increase of the percentage of the unsaturated fatty acids responsible for the membranes' fluidity. Also, timol, carvacrol, and eugenol led to an increase of the saturated fatty acid C_{16} and C_{18} concentration and to a decrease of the production of the unsaturated C_{18} fatty acids [16].

The inhibition of protein activity, which has as a consequence the perturbation of the cellular division (cinnamaldehyde, timol, eugenol, carvacrol). Timolol can also affect the expression of the proteins involved in the energetic metabolism [15].

The effect on the production of ATP and ATPase. The production of ATP in prokaryotes takes place in the cellular wall and in the cytosol through glycolysis. The volatile oils perturb the cellular membrane and modify the intracellular and extracellular ATP balance, so the ATP is lost through the disorganized membrane. This effect has been seen to be induced by terpenes with phenolic structure in the *E.*[i] *coli* and *L. monocytogenes* strains [15].

The effect on the microbial metabolism. The intracellular and extracellular metabolome presents many fundamental advantages through which this can provide important information about the functional genomics, metabolic engineering, the characterization of the strains, and mechanism of cellular communication. The microbial metabolites can change depending on the weather conditions. Recently, many powerful analytical standard approaches, including NMR, microarray, GC-MS, and LC-MS, have been used to analyze the metabolome of the bacteria under stress. These techniques are more widely used to investigate the metabolic effects of natural molecules with bacteriostatic and/or bactericidal activity [15].

The impairing of the cellular morphology. The activity of the volatile oils and of its components differs according to the form of the bacteria studied, so there was a report that bacilli are more susceptible to volatile oils than cocci. For some strains of *S. typhimurium* and *E. coli*, which have a bacillary form with a smooth surface, respectively, those of *M. luteus* and *S. aureus*, which have a normal coccoidal form, after 24 h of treatment with mint volatile oil, the cellular lesions in bacilli were more pronounced compared to cocci [15].

The quorum sensing inhibitory activity. In this regard, the volatile oils can represent the biggest available reservoir of new therapeutic agents. Bacterial QS can be inhibited through different mechanisms, including (1) inhibition of the AHL synthesis, (2) inhibition of the transport and of the AHL secretion, (3) AHL antagonist action, (4) sequestration of AHL, and (5) inhibition of downstream targets of the binding receptor of AHL. Different volatile oils extracted from ornamental plants have proven efficient against biofilms formed by *Salmonella* sp., *Listeria* sp., *Pseudomonas* sp., *Staphylococcus* sp., and *Lactobacillus* sp., demonstrating their interference with the quorum sensing mechanism, which plays a pivotal role in biofilm development [17].

2.1.2. The anti-inflammatory activity of volatile oils

The *Ocimum sanctum, Baphia nitida, Aloe barbadensis, Illicium verum, Citrus aurantium, Cinnamomum zeylanicum, Juniperus communis, Cananga odorata*, as well as eucalypt, mint, rosemary, lavender, pine, and clove volatile oils are known for their anti-inflammatory activity. This activity is mediated through multiple mechanisms, such as the inhibition of lipoxygenase, prevention of leukotriene synthesis, inhibition of COX-2 enzyme, inhibition of the pro-inflammatory cytokines IL-1 and α tumor necrosis factor, and repression of pro-inflammatory gene expression [18].

2.1.3. The antioxidant activity of volatile oils

The free radicals and the reactive oxygen species induce the oxidation of biomolecules including proteins, amino acids, unsaturated lipids, and DNA, ultimately producing molecular modification linked to aging, atherosclerosis and cancer, Alzheimer disease, Parkinson disease, diabetes, and asthma. The human body has a defense mechanism which can neutralize the free radicals present in almost all the cells. If an imbalance between the production of free radicals and their removal through the antioxidant system of the organism occurs, it is accompanied by a phenomenon known as "oxidative stress." In this condition, an external source of antioxidants is necessary to ensure a balance between the free radicals and antioxidants [19].

The volatile oils, as natural sources of phenolic compounds, have an antioxidant activity or present the capacity to neutralize the free radicals. It was noted that volatile oils with a high content of timol, carvacrol, and α-tocopherol present a very good antioxidant activity, although still inferior to that of ascorbic acid. The antioxidant activity of volatile oils cannot be attributed only to the presence of phenolic compounds; the alcoholic monoterpenes, ketones, aldehydes, hydrocarbons, and ethers from the volatile oil composition could contribute also to the neutralization of the free radical action (neral/geranial, citronellal, izomenton, menton, α-terpinen, γ-terpinen, α-terpinolenes, linalool, and 1,8-cineol). It is obvious that the volatile oils can be considered potential natural sources of antioxidants and can be, probably, used as daily supplements or additives to prevent the oxidative stress which contributes to many degenerative diseases [19].

2.2. Plant-derived compounds

The phytochemical studies on the plant extracts are currently headed toward the isolation and identification of the components from the complex mixtures with the purpose of establishing structure-biological activity and dose-effect correlations.

Based on the chemical structure of diverse essential oils, they are divided in two large, distinct groups: (i) terpenes (monoterpenes and sesquiterpenes) and terpenoids (isoprenoid) and (ii) the group of aromatic and aliphatic compounds [20].

2.2.1. Terpenes and terpenoids

The structural diversity and the different potential biological activities of sesquiterpenes, such as anticancer, anti-inflammatory, antitumoral, antimalaria, antiviral, antibacterial, antifungal, etc., have increased the researches' interest for the discovery of new drugs [21].

2.2.2. Carotenoids and carotenes

Carotenes are pigments of leaves, fruits, and flowers with yellow shades which are localized in the chromoplasts. In the plant organism, they could be found in free state or in combination with holoproteins and carbohydrates. The content in carotenoidic pigments depends on the species nature and the influence of environment's conditions [22]. Due to the hydrocarbon chemical structure, the carotenes are hydrophobic substances, soluble only in organic solvents, oils, and fats.

2.2.3. The aglicons of phenolic heterosides

2.2.3.1. Antimicrobial activity

Currently there are only a few studies regarding the antimicrobial action of polyphenolic compounds. For flavonoids a correlation between the chemical structure and their antimicrobial properties was realized, but these compounds can target different components and functions of the bacterial cells. It was noticed that the flavanone dihydroxylated 2, 4—and 2,6—at the level of B ring and 5,7-dihydroxylated at the level of the A ring have a significantly increased antimicrobial activity. The change of the six and eight positions with an aliphatic group with a long chain, such as lavandulil or geranil, leads to an improvement of the activity. An improvement of the flavan-3-ols activity with the substitution of some aliphatic chains C8 and C10 was noted [23].

Chalcones are more efficient against *S. aureus* than flavonones or flavones, the hydroxyl in 2—position being important for the antimicrobial activity of these compounds. For methoxylated flavonoids a drastic reduction of the antibacterial activity was reported. The substitution of the B ring with the 3′-chloro, 4′-chloro, and 4′-bromo has led to an increase of the antimicrobial activity, being two times more efficient than the simple underived compound on the *S. aureus* strain and four times more active against *Enterococcus faecalis*. Also the 2′,4′-dichlor derivate presents a four to eight times improvement of the activity against the *S. aureus* strain and four times against *E. faecalis*. The 3-methyl-6-bromoflavanon compounds are less active; thus, the halogen substitution of the A ring decreases the antimicrobial activity [23].

Phenolic acids (garlic and ferulic) significantly changed the hydrophobicity and total charge of the cellular surface, as well as the secretion of K^+, leading to pore formation in the cellular membrane of both gram-positive and gram-negative microorganisms [24].

According to Cueva et al. [25], the number and position of the substituents in the benzenic nucleus from the phenolic acid structure and the length of the lateral saturated chains influence in different ways the antimicrobial potential. The antimicrobial activity for different polyphenolic acids decreased in the following order: 4-hydroxy- >> 3-hydroxy- > 4-hydroxy-3-metoxy- > 3,4-dihydroxy- > unsubstituted benzoic acids. For phenylacetic acids, the order of antimicrobial activity was unsubstituted> 3-hydroxy- > 4-hydroxy- >substituted 3,4-dihydroxy, while for phenylpropionic acids, the order was unsubstituted> 4-hydroxy > 3-hydroxy > 3,4-dihydroxy [25].

The potential mechanism of action of the polyphenolic components:

- *The inhibition of nucleic acid synthesis*: the low concentration of polyphenols affects the activity of energy production-associated enzymes, while the high concentration has determined the protein precipitation. In a study using radioactive precursors, it was shown that the DNA synthesis was strongly inhibited in *Proteus vulgaris*, while the mRNA synthesis was most affected in the *S. aureus* strain. The polyphenolic compounds which present this activity have been robinetin, myricetin, and (−)-epigallocatechin [26].
- *The perturbation of the cytoplasmatic membrane*. Phenols can interact with the phospholipidic component from the cellular membrane increasing the cellular membrane permeability or causing significant modification of the fatty acid composition and phospholipids in the structure of the microbial membrane. For the phenolic compounds, it was proven that they can cause rapid swelling of the *P. aeruginosa* cells [27]. The effect on the cytoplasmatic membrane integrity of *S. aureus* was investigated also by measuring the intracellular potassium loss, observing an approximately 20 % loss comparing with the untreated cells with the studied phenolic compound. These data suggest that in the cytoplasmatic membrane, lesions are induced leading to the leak of intracellular potassium [23].
- *Inhibition of energetic metabolism*. It is well known that BHA, p-cumaric, and caffeic acids attack not only the cytoplasmatic membrane, perturbing the permeability and leading to intracellular constituent release, but also affecting the membrane functions responsible for electron transport, nutrient absorption, nucleic acid synthesis, and ATPase activity; in other words the bactericidal/bacteriostatic effect of phenolic compounds is the result of damages at two levels, i.e., the membrane and the cell wall integrity and the physiological state of bacterial cells [28].

Plaper et al. [29] have reported that quercetin binds to the GyrB unit of the DNA-gyrase of *E. coli* and inhibits the ATPase enzyme's activity. The flavonoids' binding site was bunked over those of ATP and novobiocin (antibiotic that blocks replication), because of the adding of these compounds which have interfered with the quercetin's fluorescence [23].

2.2.3.2. Immunomodulatory activity of polyphenolic compounds

The inflammation is the host's response to the invasion of a foreign body, such as infectious agents or inert foreign bodies. In this context, the inflammatory response is an acute protection reaction triggered in the course of irritation, lesions, or infections, characterized by erythema, heat, edema, and pain clinical signs. The redness and the heat result from a blood flux increase; the edema is associated with increased vascular permeability and plasma extravasation. The edema is pressing on the afferent endings of nerve fibers, leading to the appearance of the pain sensation, to which also contribute the small-size polypeptidic molecules called kinins. In normal conditions, these changes in the inflamed tissue serve to isolate and limit the negative effects on the organism [30]. The most secondary metabolites of plants such as phenolic acids, flavonoids, iridoids, monoterpenoids, and triterpenoids are known for their capacity to intervene directly or indirectly, in the following mechanisms: production of inflammatory mediators (metabolites of arachnoid acid (AA), peptides, cytokines, excitators or amino acids, etc.); the production and/or the activity of messengers (cGMP, cAMP), different protein kinases, and calcium; modification of the expression of the transcription factors, such as AP-1, NFkB, and proto-oncogenes (c-jun, c-fos, and c-myc); and the expression of key pro-inflammatory molecules, such as the NO synthase (iNOS), cyclooxygenase (COX-2), cytokines (IL-1β, TNF-α, etc.), neuropeptides, and proteases [30, 31].

2.2.3.3. The inhibition of the arachnoid acid pathway by polyphenolic compounds

One of the most important anti-inflammatory mechanisms is the inhibition of phospholipase A_2, cyclooxygenase, and lipoxygenase enzymes, thus reducing the prostaglandins (PGs) and leukotrienes concentration [32]. The arachnoid acid (AA) is released from membranary phospholipids by phospholipase A_2 cleavage (PLA_2), and it can be metabolized by cyclooxygenase pathway (COX) in prostaglandins (PGs) and thromboxane A_2 (TXA_2) or through the lipoxygenase pathway (LOX) in the hydroperoxyeicosatetraenoic (HpETEs) and hydroxyeicosatetraenoic (HETEs) acids and leukotrienes (LTs) [33]. Cyclooxygenase exists in two major isoforms (COX-1, COX-2) and a variety COX-3 [34]. COX-1 is expressed in many tissues, while COX-2 is known as an inducible enzyme which produces, in many cases, important quantities of prostanglandins. COX-2 is strongly expressed in inflammatory cells, which include macrophages and mast cells, after the stimulation with pro-inflammatory cytokines and/or lipopolysaccharides (LPS) [35]. LOXs are enzymes that participate in the formation of hydroxyl acids and leukotrienes from the arachnoid acid. The most known are metabolites resulted from the action of 5-lipoxygenase, an enzyme present especially in neutrophils. 5- and 12-LOXs produce 5-HETE and 12-HETE, which induce an inflammatory response. Prostaglandins and leukotrienes are present in the inflammatory exudate, and the agents that inhibit the cyclooxygenase exhibit an in vivo anti-inflammatory action [36].

The polyphenolic compounds have proven to inhibit the cellular enzymes, such as PLA_2, COX, and LOX, with the purpose to reduce the production of arachnoid acid, prostaglandins, and leukotrienes, thus exerting the anti-inflammatory action [33]. The polyphenolic compounds extracted from red wine and black tea have been capable to modulate the COX-2 activity and the genes' expression in different cell types [37]. For example, quercetin has reduced the mRNA expression of COX-2 in the Caco2 cells stimulated by IL-1β but also in unstimulated cells [38], in the peritoneal leukocytes of the rat [39] and in the guinea pig epiderma [40]. After the treatment of rabbit's articular chondrocytes with resveratrol, it was noted that the expression levels of cyclooxygenase (COX-2) and prostaglandin E2 (PGE2) have began to increase in 10 min, reaching maximal levels after 3 h, and then they began to decrease. Also, it was demonstrated that resveratrol provokes the phosphorylation of mitogen-activated protein kinases and Akt from rabbit's articular chondrocytes. The inhibition of mitogen-activated protein kinases and Akt with PD98059, SB203580, LY294002, and triciribin by resveratrol has led to the suppression of type II collagen induction and COX-2 expression [41]. It has been reported that other polyphenols from green tea, namely, prodelphinidin B-4,3′-O-galat and prodelphinidin B2 3,3′-di-O-galat, have the capacity to suppress mRNA, the COX-2 expression protein, and the release of PGE_2 in a dose-dependent manner. Moreover, (−)-epigallocatechin (EGC), (−)-gallocatechin (GC), galat-(−)-epicatechin (ECG), galat-(−)-catechin(CG), and galat-(−)-epigallocatechin (EGCG) have proven to have an inhibitory activity on COX-1/COX-2 for different human and mouse cell lines [42]. Also, kaempferol, a flavonoid present in different superior plants, has decreased significantly the production of PGE_2 by LPS stimulation of human cells in the culture whole blood [43].

Tirozol, lycopene, and quercetin have inhibited the COX-2 and iNOS gene expression in RAW 264.7 macrophages stimulated in association with interferon-γ (IFN-γ), probably through NFkB pathway. These data suggest that these compounds can act as nontoxic agents by the control of pro-inflammatory genes involved in celiac disease [42].

2.2.3.4. Modulating cytokine production

Cytokines are the main local mediators of intercellular communication necessary for an integrated response to a variety of stimuli in the course of immune and inflammatory response [32]. Many cytokines have been identified in tissues in a series of inflammatory diseases with immunological substrate. More than that, a "balance" between the pro-inflammatory effects (IL-1β, IL-2, TNF-α, IL-6, and IFN-γ) and anti-inflammatory cytokines (IL-8, IL-10, IL-4, TGFβ) is considered a determinant factor in the disease evolution [42]. For this reason, the modulation of the cytokine profile represents an interesting objective for the development of anti-inflammatory drugs useful in the clinical practice. The polyphenolic compounds, which can interfere selectively with the production or/and function of cytokines, can offer an important alternative for the treatment of many inflammatory diseases [44]. With this purpose, it was observed that many polyphenolic compounds are capable to reduce the expression of different pro-inflammatory cytokines/chemokines, such as TNF-α, IL-1β, IL-6, and MCP-1, in many cell types, such as monocytes stimulated with phorbol-12-myristate-13-acetate (PMA) or phytohemagglutinin (PHA) [44], human activated astrocytes [45], human synovial cells [46], the human cellular line of activate mast cells, CMH-1 stimulated with calcium ionophore A23187 (PMACI) [47], fibroblasts of nasal mucosa, and bronchial epithelial cells A549 [48].

These studies sustain the fact that polyphenols have the capacity to modulate the immune answer through their anti-inflammatory potential [49]. However, the effects on the balance between the pro-inflammatory and anti-inflammatory cytokines have proven to be specific depending on the chemical structure of polyphenols [42]. The anti-inflammatory mechanism of quercetin consists in the inhibition of the expression of pro-inflammatory cytokines in the mast cell and in suppression of TNF-α [50].

2.2.3.5. The modulation of NFkB-dependent signaling pathways

From their discovery the transcription factors NFkB/Rel are considered responsible for chronic and acute inflammatory diseases. NFkB plays an essential role in the trigger of the inflammatory, stress, proliferative, and apoptotic responses [51]. NFkB coordinates the induction of a wide area of genes which encode the pro-inflammatory cytokines (IL-1, IL-2, IL-6, and TNF-α); chemokines (MIP-1α and MCP-1); cellular adhesion molecules (ICAM, VCAM, E-selectin); acute phase proteins; immune receptors; growth factors; inducible enzymes such as the growth factor of vascular endothelium (VEGF), COX-2, matrix metalloproteinase (MMP), and iNOS; and all the molecules involved in inflammation, cellular proliferation, cellular adhesion, migration, and invasion [52]. The inhibition of NFkB is generally considered a useful strategy in the treatment of inflammatory disturbances [51], this pathway being an important and attractive therapeutic target. It was observed that plant polyphenols can act as modulators of transduction pathways of the signal to trigger their beneficial effects [53]. The NFkB/Rel family is formed by five members: p65 (RelA), RelB, c-Rel, p50/p105 (NFκB1), and p52/p100 (NFκB2), these being DNA-binding proteins which recognize a common sequence [54]. In unstimulated cells, NFkB is sequestered in the cytoplasm in inactive form [55]. Polyphenols have proven to present an anti-inflammatory activity by modulating the NFkB activity. Through the influence of (−)-epigallocatechin galat polyphenolic component on the NFkB pathway, the inhibitory effect of this compound was demonstrated by counteracting IKK activation and IκBα degradation [42].

Flavonoids present the capacity to modulate the activation cascade of NFkB [56]. In RAW 264.7 cells activated with IFNγ, quercetin, tirozol, and lycopene have inhibited the iNOS, COX-2 expression, and pro-inflammatory genes, by the prevention of nuclear translocation of the subunits p50 and p65 of NFkB, STAT-1α, and IRF-1. These results suggest that lycopene, quercetin, and tirozol can be potential nontoxic agents in the control of bowel inflammation in the celiac disease trough the prevention of the activation of the signaling pathway of transduction [57]. The beneficial anti-inflammatory effects exhibited by quercetin, in vitro and in vivo, seem to be due to the inhibition of the phosphorylation protein IκBα, which, through the blocking of the NFkN pathway, leads to the counteraction of the cytokine expression and the induction of oxide nitric synthesis [44]. In a similar way, in the human mast cell line, quercetin has led to the decrease in the pro-inflammatory cytokine expression (TNF-α, IL-1β, IL-6) and anti-inflammatory cytokine expression (IL-8) through the degradation of IκBα and nuclear translocation of p65, blocking the activation of NFkB [47].

2.3. Propolis

Propolis, the so-called bee glue, is a natural product of double origin: vegetal and animal. Thus, the bees elaborate this product by adding glandular secretions and wax to the resinous substances collected from different species of plants. Besides its mechanical purpose (sealing the holes and cracks, limiting the entry in the hive, reparations of the honeycombs), propolis has an antiseptic role in the hive's microclimate, being a real "chemical weapon" against the microorganisms [58, 59].

Since ancient times, propolis has been used in folk medicine, being one of the most efficient natural remedies. The active pharmacological compounds from propolis are present in variable quantities depending on the propolis sample, the way of dosing, and the nature of the extraction method [60]. The ratio of the organic compounds in propolis is very important for determining the biological effects [59]. The main constituents of propolis are phenolic compounds (flavonoids, phenolic acids, and their esters), aromatic acids, aliphatic acids and their esters, terpenoids, and bioactive compounds responsible for the biologic effect of propolis [61]. Flavonoids are considered to be responsible for the main therapeutic actions of propolis. It has been proven that the anti-infectious effects of propolis are different depending on the geographic area, botanical origin, and microbial species on which they act. Besides the therapeutic efficiency manifested in different diseases, propolis exercises also an immunomodulating action with an important role on the stimulation of the organism's capacity of defense. On an international level, the studies performed in some well-known pharmacology and medicine laboratories have confirmed the special role that this product plays for the human organism in the prophylaxis and the treatment of a wide variety of afflictions. In the natural state or in the extracted form, tinctures, and different pharmaceutical forms, propolis represents at this time one of the most important points of interest for the study and work of apitherapy. The international research has demonstrated that at the associated use with some antibiotics, the efficacy and length of action of the propolis extract are stressed and the studied microorganisms do not develop resistance to antibiotics. Due to the multiple chemical components, propolis is considered the most valuable bee product, with a wide variety of therapeutic actions: bactericidal, antiseptic, antiparasitic, antiviral, antioxidant, wound healing, anti-inflammatory, analgesic, antitumoral, regenerative, and immunomodulatory [62].

Many plants or plant-derived compounds with high levels of antioxidant properties also manifest wound-healing benefits. There are several studies that document the use of plant extracts in the development of bioactive wound dressings.

3. Plant extracts used in wound management

3.1. Essential oils

Oil extracts are widely used in skin care and treatment. A couple of oil extracts have proven antibacterial activities: oleo-gum-resin of *Commiphora guidotti* Chiov. ex. Guid. [63]; *Copaifera officinalis* and *Pentaclethra macroloba* [64], and the oily extract of *Rosa damascena* petals in combination with aqueous extracts of *Malva sylvestris* and *Solanum nigrum* leaves [65] (against *Staphylococcus aureus*). *Calophyllum inophyllum* L showed antibacterial activity against gram-positive bacteria by direct inhibition of mitotic growth and against gram-negative bacteria due to increased release of β-defensin 2 peptide by macrophages [66]. Moreover, the two Amazonian plants,

Copaifera officinalis and *Pentaclethra macroloba,* have proved well-documented anti-inflammatory, antimicrobial, emollient, moisturizing, and wound-healing activities [64]. An extracted oil from pumpkin seeds (*Cucurbita pepo* L.) can be a promising drug for healing wounds in animal studies (uniform wounds induced on the dorsum of rats) due to a high content of polyunsaturated fatty acids (linoleic acid, 50.88 ± 0.106 g/100 g of total fatty acids), tocopherols (280 ppm), and sterols (2086.5 ± 19.092 ppm) [67]. Several oil extracts have been successfully tried in burn wound models in rats. A poly-herbal cream containing aqueous extracts of *Malva sylvestris* and *Solanum nigrum* leaves and oily extracts of *Rosa damascena* petals, retrieved from Iranian traditional medicine, showed desirable reepithelialization with remarkable neovascularization with less inflammatory cells [65]. The oil extracted from the seeds of *Calophyllum inophyllum* L. (Calophyllaceae), an evergreen tree ethnomedically used along the seashores and islands of the Indian and Pacific Oceans, especially in Polynesia is traditionally used topically to treat a wide range of skin injuries from burn, scar, and infected wounds. The human keratinocyte cells were used to test the safety profile and wound-healing properties of the *Calophyllum inophyllum* L and proved efficient and safe in wound healing [66]. The oil extract (BBO) obtained from *Blumea balsamifera* (L.) DC (ainaxiang) was tested in deep second-degree burn model in rats. The plasma levels of interleukin-1 (IL-1) and tumor necrosis factor-alpha (TNF-α) decreased, but the tissue expressions of basic fibroblast growth factor (bFGF), vascular endothelial growth factor (VEGF), and transforming growth factor-beta (TGF-β) increased, so the healing accelerated after treatment with BBO in the burn injury rats [68].

3.2. *Calendula officinalis*

Marigold (*Calendula officinalis*) is an annual culture plant species, part of the daisy family (Asteraceae), rarely biannual, 40–80 cm tall, with a powerful balsamic scent [69, 70].

The *Calendula officinalis* extract contains different classes of compounds, such as triterpenoids, flavonoids, coumarins, quinones, volatile oil, carotenoids, and amino acids [71], but the active compound consists mainly of carotenoids (carotene, lycopene, flavoxanthin, lutein, and rubixanthin) and faradiol [72].

It is widely used in Romania as a universal, wonder cream. Many patients use it for its anti-inflammatory, anticancer, antibacterial, antifungal, antiviral, and wound-healing activity [71, 73, 74]. It is used in clinical applications such as wounds, leg ulcers, first-degree burns, contusions, and skin rashes (acute dermatitis during breast cancer treatment) [71, 75].

A study tried to link the angiogenic activity of *Calendula officinalis* L. grown in Brazil to the expression of VEGF but without success and suggested that maybe it is due to other pro-angiogenic factors (fibroblast growth factors (FGF) or angiogenic cytokines (interleukin-8 (IL-8), tumor necrosis factor-alpha (TNF-α), and transforming growth factor-β (TGF-β)) [76].

Studies on effects of *C. officinalis* tincture (CDOT) on cell viability and wound closure proved that it stimulated both proliferation and migration of fibroblasts in a statistically significant manner; in a PI3K-dependent pathway, the identified compounds are likely to be responsible for wound-healing activity [71]. Additionally, homeopathic preparations composed of *Arnica montana, C. officinalis, H. perforatum,* and *Symphytum officinale* have been shown to promote proliferation and migration of NIH-3T3 fibroblast cells [71].

Another preparation using marigold was designed for treating chronic ocular surface diseases. A formulation consisting of solid lipid nanoparticles (SLN), long-chain fatty acids (palmitic acid, stearic acid, or arachidic acid), Epikuron 200 (purified phosphatidylcholine), and bile salts (cholate, taurocholate, or taurodeoxycholate) has been prepared by dilution of a microemulsion. Then it was loaded with *Calendula officinalis* extract. Calendula-loaded SLN were nontoxic, with a good stability and a good lyophilization profile, probably useful for prolonged storage conditions [72].

3.3. Aloe vera

Aloe vera is a cactus-like plant [77] that belongs to Liliaceae family [78], originated in South Africa [79]. It has been shown to have benefits when used to accelerate wound healing [78].

There have been more than 75 active ingredients including aloesin, aloe emodin, acemannan, aloeride, methylchromones, flavonoids, saponin, amino acids, vitamins, and minerals [80].

The whole gel extract of aloe vera has been reported to promote wound, burn, and frost-bite healing, in addition to having anti-inflammatory, strong immunomodulatory and large spectrum antibacterial (*Staphylococcus aureus, Escherichia coli, Pseudomonas aeruginosa, Salmonella typhi, S. pyogenes, S. mutans, A. actinomycetemcomitans, P. gingivalis, B. fragilis, Enterococcus bovis, A. hydrophila, Salmonella paratyphi, Bacillus subtilis, H. pylori*), antifungal (*Candida parapsilosis, Candida krusei, Candida albicans*), antiviral (herpes simplex virus type 2 strain, encephalomyocarditis virus, influenza A) activity, hypoglycemic, hepatoprotective effect, gastroprotective properties, laxative effects, antihyperlipidemic activity, and anti-aging effect [79, 81, 82]. Its healing property is related to a compound that is called glucomannan [78]. The mannose-6-phosphate increases wound contraction and collagen synthesis [79]. β-Sitosterol (found in aloe vera mucilage) increases angiogenesis and promotes a better healing of traumatic tissues by increasing the rate of genetic expression of VEGF and its receptor in the wound tissue [78]. The known targets and effects of available topical treatments in the processes of wound healing, skin scarring, and abnormal raised dermal scarring such as keloid and hypertrophic scarring are soothing/anti-inflammatory effect, hydration and moisturisation, and improved skin/scar condition [83].

In 1990 the efficacy of aloe vera saturated polyethylene oxide (PEO) dressings for treating full-face dermabrasion wounds was proven [81]. An amorphous hydrogel dressing derived from the aloe plant (Carrasyn Gel Wound Dressing, Carrington Laboratories, Inc., Irving, TX) has been approved by the Food and Drug Administration for the management of Stages I through IV pressure ulcers being as effective as a moist saline gauze wound dressing [84]. A couple of studies performed by Silva et al. included sodium alginate/polyvinyl alcohol films loaded with aloe vera and vitamin E, capable of enhancing healing in burn wounds [81], and blended membranes composed of chitosan (CTS) and aloe vera gel, cross-linked with genipin to improve their properties (in vitro cell culture studies evidenced that the L929 cells have high cell viability) [85]. Another study on mice with burn wounds demonstrated the healing properties of aloe emodin in combination with resveratrol, without a cytotoxic to THP-1 macrophages [86]. Moreover a dressing film comprising 1.95 % w/v fibroin and 0.05 % w/v aloe gel [87] and an aloe vera-olive oil combination cream may find application in treatment of diabetic nonhealing skin ulcers [88]. Another bioactive dressing was designed using collagen-chitosan scaffolds supplemented with aloe vera [81].

3.4. Curcumin

Curcumin, a natural yellow phenolic antioxidant compound, is present in many kinds of herbs, particularly in *Curcuma longa* Linn. (turmeric), the main curcuminoid present in turmeric [89, 90].

It contains methoxy groups and phenols, which are responsible for its biological and pharmacological properties, being shown to possess significant anti-inflammatory, antioxidant, anticarcinogenic, anti-mutagenic, anticoagulant, and anti-infective effects [89, 91]. Curcumin has hepatoprotective, nephroprotective, cardioprotective, neuroprotective, anticancer, hypoglycemic, antirheumatic, and antidiabetic activities, and it also suppresses thrombosis and protects against myocardial infarction and treats many diseases including cough, rheumatism, diabetes, biliary disorders, anorexia, sinusitis, hepatic disorders, cancer, and Alzheimer disease [90, 92].

Curcumin has been used for wound healing [89] because of the anti-inflammatory activity due to the inhibition of TNF-α, COX-2, STAT, cyclin D1, NFkB signaling pathways; IL-1b, IL-8, IL-6 expressions; downregulation of the expression of MMP-8, and acute phase proteins [93]. Also the wound-healing potential of curcumin is attributed to its anti-infectious and antioxidant properties [89]. Curcumin is involved in tissue remodeling, granulation tissue formation, and collagen deposition and increases fibroblast proliferation and vascular density [89].

Moreover two new synthetic analogs of curcumin (C66 and B06) proved to reduce TNF-α and NO production; downregulated mRNA levels of IL-1b, TNF-k, IL-6, IL-12, COX-2, as well as iNOS; and prevented activation of JNK/NFkB signaling in high glucose stimulated primary peritoneal macrophages [93].

The antibacterial activity of curcumin is due to its action against the bacterial membrane [94]. Curcumin inhibited the growth of periodontopathic bacteria *P. gingivalis, Prevotella intermedia, Fusobacterium nucleatum, Treponema denticola* [95], foodborne bacteria *Bacillus cereus* and *Escherichia coli* [96], methicillin-resistant *Staphylococcus aureus* (*MRSA*) [97], *Enterococcus faecalis, Bacillus subtilis, Streptococcus mutants*, and *Pseudomonas aeruginosa* [94].

Curcumin has been used in different nanoformulations used to increased solubilization of curcumin but at the same time protect curcumin against inactivation by hydrolysis: liposomes, polymeric nanoparticles, polymeric micelles, conjugates, peptide/protein carriers, cyclodextrins, solid dispersions, etc. However, most nanoformulations are administered parenterally [90].

The compound glucosyl-THC increased the epithelialization and granulation tissue formation, with nonstaining, nontoxic, nonirritant, and non-skin-sensitive side effects. Thus the synthesized glucosyl-THC may act as a promising therapeutic agent in the future, in the management of excision wounds, and in cosmetic applications [98].

Curcumin has demonstrated its efficacy for healing of diabetic wound in a work that used curcumin (Cur)-loaded poly(-caprolactone) (PCL)/gum tragacanth (GT) scaffold membranes fabricated by electrospinning. The scaffold membranes obtained a controlled release of curcumin for over 20 days [92]. Another design implied chitosan (CTS)/chondroitin sulfate (CS) nanoparticles, both pure and curcumin-loaded, synthesized by ionic gelation, investigated as a way to reduce the viability of human lung tumor cells [91].

To enhance the properties of curcumin, it has been combined with ginger, and the two were dissolved in dimethyl sulfoxide. A 500 μl of solutions containing 10 % curcumin, 3 % ginger extract, and topical dermatocorticoid were used as pretreatment on hairless rats. The pretreatment improved healing of subsequently induced abrasion skin wound-treated rats, maybe because the ginger extract increases vascularity and blood flow in the repairing tissue, while curcumin acts on matrix remodeling. Still, we should not overlook the anti-inflammatory properties of dermatocorticosteroids [99].

On the other hand, a cellular biomechanics approach where automated quantitative wound-healing assays were used did not identify significant effects of curcumin, aloe vera, and ginger on en-mass migration kinematics of fibroblasts in damaged cultures [100].

3.5. Other plant species used in wound healing

Many Brazilian plants have proven efficient in wound healing. *Struthanthus vulgaris*, *H. speciosa* leaves Gomes (Apocynaceae), *Casearia sylvestris* Sw. (popularly known as guaçatonga), *Achyrocline satureioid*es DC Lam., *Matricaria recutita* L., *Melia azedarach* L., and *Mirabilis jalapa* L. are the most recently evaluated, usually on fibroblasts, keratinocytes, and rats. The aqueous extracts from these plants demonstrated the ability to stimulate keratinocytes' growth up and also fibroblast proliferation resulting in a positive cell proliferation [101]. In an experimental wound model in rats, *Struthanthus vulgaris*, in a 5 % ointment, was capable of modulating the release of pro- and anti-inflammatory cytokines (IL-1α, TNF-α and IL-10, nitric oxide, and growth factors such as TGF-β), improving the quality of the scar tissue [102]. Also the ethanolic extract of *H. speciosa* leaves Gomes (Apocynaceae) demonstrated its effects on the release of the pro-inflammatory cytokine tumor necrosis factor (TNF-α) by lipopolysaccharide (LPS)-stimulated human acute monocytic (THP-1) cells. Moreover, *H. speciosa* showed an increase cell migration and proliferation of fibroblasts compared with control cells, as well as a reduced TNF-α release by LPS-stimulated THP-1 cells. All together, the results indicate that it can be used to treat wounds and inflammatory disorders [103]. Another hydroalcoholic extract of *Casearia sylvestris* Sw. showed benefits in the treatment of inflammatory conditions, in second-degree scald burn injuries, and in an experimental wound model, most likely due to its analgesic, antiseptic, and anti-inflammatory activities [104].

Traditional Turkish medicine has many important plants used to treat ulcers, burns, and wounds. *Hypericum perforatum* (HP) (St. John's Wort-Kantaron), widely for the treatment of burn injuries for many years in traditional Turkish medicine, was compared with silver sulfadiazine (SS) in the treatment of second-degree thermal burn created on the dorsal sites of rats. The measures of epidermal thickness and number of vessels demonstrated that HP administered four times a day within the first 24 h is clearly effective in wound healing in the experimental thermal second-degree burn and is significantly superior to SS treatment [105]. The roots and root barks of *Echium* sp. (*E. italicum* L, *E. vulgare* L., and *E. angustifolium*) have been also used to treat ulcers, burns, and wounds in traditional Turkish medicine. Thus an experimental study using ethanol root extract of *Echium* sp. on linear incision experimental models showed remarkable wound-healing activity [106]. Three species—*A. coarctata* Poir. (AC), *A. kotschyi* Boiss. subsp. *kotschyi* (AK), and *A. lycaonica* Boiss. and Heldr. (AL) (genus *Achillea* L.)—were evaluated for their phenolic compositions, total phenolic contents, antioxidant properties, wound-healing potencies on NIH-3T3 fibroblasts, and cytotoxic effects on MCF-7 human breast cancer cells. AK was the most valuable source of flavonoids and chlorogenic acid with important antioxidant, wound-healing, and cytotoxic activities [107].

Various plant parts including leaves, fruits, stem bark, and root extracts of 61 African medicinal plants belonging to 36 families were reported to have scientifically demonstrated wound-healing properties [108]. Widely used in Ethiopia for treatment of wound, *Rumex abyssinicus* Jacq (Polygonaceae) has been evaluated as ointment (an extraction of the rhizomes of the plant with 80 % methanol) on an excision model in mice. The hydroalcoholic extract increased wound contraction, shortened the epithelization time, increased the hydroxyproline content, and also reduced the inflammation [109]. A hydroalcoholic leaf extract of *Combretum mucronatum*, a medicinal plant widely used in West African traditional medicine, proved beneficial effects for wound-healing and anthelmintic activity [110].

A herbal ointment containing 10 % *Salvadora persica* extract was compared with Solcoseryl jelly 10 % and blank Vaseline using excision wound-healing model in animals. The 10 % *Salvadora persica* extract and 10 % Solcoseryl jelly showed superiority in the acceleration rate of wound enclosure in rats [111].

The ethanolic extract of the bark of *Calotropis procera* was evaluated for the antioxidant potential and the wound-healing effect using excision and incision wound on normal and dexamethasone-suppressed wound-healing rodent models. It revealed a potential wound-healing agent due to improved collagen deposition and reduced inflammatory reaction [112, 113].

Moringa oleifera (MO), another herb used as a traditional folk medicine for the management of wound healing and associated conditions, has proven its efficacy by promoting fibroblast proliferation and migration through increasing the wound closure rate corroborating its traditional use [114].

Polygonum aviculare L. with ingredients such as quercitrin hydrate, caffeic acid, and rutin has been known for its antioxidant and anti-obesity effects. Moreover it accelerated the motility of HaCaT keratinocytes with the activation of Wnt/β-catenin signaling, without showing significant leading to efficiently reepithelized wounds generated on mice [115].

An extract of the leaves of *Porophyllum ruderale* and laser irradiation on the healing of burns were effective in decreasing the granulocytes during the repair process indicating a possible anti-inflammatory action of this extract of native flora [116].

Allium ascalonicum Linn., commonly called shallot, have been reported to be beneficial in wound healing due to its antibacterial (inhibiting the gram-positive *Staphylococcus epidermidis* and *Bacillus subtilis* ATCC 6633 strains) and antioxidant properties [117] on wound models in rats.

Ampelopsis radix has been used as a traditional Korean medicine for the treatment of burns and scalds. The healing effect of *A. japonica* root tuber ethanol extract (AJE) was shown on induced cutaneous scald injury in Sprague Dawley (SD) rats, by decreasing the TNF-α and TGF-β1 levels and increasing the IL-10 levels [118].

The methanol extract of *Rubus ellipticus* leaves showed antioxidant activity and antitumor and wound-healing properties in incision, excision, and *Staphylococcus aureus*-induced-infected wound models and mice with Ehrlich ascites carcinoma [119].

A 10 % gel of unripe banana (*Musa sapientum*) peel used in treating surgical wounds in rats proved anti-inflammatory activity (the presence of mononuclear cells and the decreased presence of polymorphonuclear cells), fibroblast proliferation, so stimulated wound healing [120].

Broken rice maltodextrin showed better functionality properties than other maltodextrin sources with a beneficial role in wound healing due to its ability to proliferate the NIH 3T3 fibroblast-wounded cells without causing cytotoxic effect [121].

3.6. Propolis

Well known from ancient times as a remedy for disease, propolis is a complex resinous mixture collected by bees from exudates of plants, with high medicinal value [122, 123].

There are three possible sources for the organic compounds of propolis: plants, secreted substances from honeybee metabolism, and materials that are introduced during propolis formation [122].

Propolis is found in many parts of the world (Europe, North America, New Zealand, and temperate zones of Asia, Brazil (green and red propolis), Russia, Cuba, Venezuela, etc.). Based on physicochemical properties such as color, texture, chemical composition, and geographic origin, Brazilian propolis is classified into 13 types [123].

Propolis contains more than 180 separate compounds (typically 50 % resin and vegetable balsam, 30 % wax, 10 % essential and aromatic oils, 5 % pollen, and 5% other substances), and while its ingredients differ based on plants in different geographic regions accessed by propolis-making bees, the main active components are thought to be present in all forms of propolis [122, 124]. Although caffeic acid phenethyl ester (CAPE) and flavonoids are characteristic constituents of poplar-type propolis, the typical constituents of Brazilian green propolis (from *Baccharis dracunculifolia*) are caffeoylquinic and prenylated cinnamic acids, such as artepillin C and baccharin [125]. Since the content of flavonoid found in the red propolis extracts was higher than that observed in the green ones [126].

Propolis has antioxidant and anti-inflammatory activity. The flavonoids and caffeic acid phenyl ester (CAPE) concentrated in propolis are powerful antioxidants [127] increasing the cellular immune response through the increase of mRNA synthesis for interferon-γ, activation of the production of other cytokines [128], and scavenging free radicals [125]. The anti-inflammatory activity has been attributed to the presence of active flavonoids (acacetin, quercetin, and naringenin) and cinnamic acid derivatives (caffeic acid phenyl ester (CAPE) and caffeic acid (CA)).CAPE and galangin, both being typical poplar propolis constituents, exhibited anti-inflammatory activity and significantly inhibited carrageenan oedema, carrageenan pleurisy, and adjuvant arthritis inflammations in rats. Dietary propolis significantly suppressed the lipoxygenase pathway of arachidonic acid metabolism during inflammation in vivo. CAPE was a more potent modulator of arachidonic acid metabolism than caffeic acid, quercetin, and naringenin [128]. CAPE, a polyphenolic compound, with cytoprotective activities and protective effects enhanced the closure of diabetic wounds and decreased the levels of IL-1β, IL-6, TNF-α, and MMP9 [124, 127]. A study on diabetic mice with leg wounds showed that the protease MMP-9 in wound fluid has importance as a marker of foot ulcer healing in diabetes. High levels of active MMP-9 correlates with poor wound healing [124]. Propolis significantly enhanced the production of collagen via the TGF-β1/Smad 2,3 signaling axis in wounded tissues [129]. Brazilian green propolis (from *Baccharis dracunculifolia*) can suppress an important inflammatory component (cell influx) and reduces the vascular permeability, angiogenesis without compromising the repair process by reducing fibrosis and increasing the pro-inflammatory markers and cytokine (TNF-α) involved in fibrinolytic activity [125, 130]. Moreover, propolis has been used in combination with honey in a synergistic effect for wound healing [131], maybe due to the honey's hydrogen peroxide, high osmolality, acidity, non-peroxide factors, nitric oxide, and phenols [132].

The mechanism of antimicrobial activity of propolis is complex and could be attributed to the synergistic activity between phenolic and other compounds, mainly to the flavonoids, pinocembrin, galangin, and pinobanksin pinocembrin, pinobanksin, p-coumaric acid benzylester, and caffeic acid phenethyl ester (CAPE) [126, 128].

Many studies showed the antibacterial activity of propolis on *Staphylococcus aureus* [133], *Staphylococcus epidermidis, Micrococcus glutamicus, Bacillus subtilis, Pseudomonas aeruginosa, Streptococcus pyogenes, Streptococcus mutans, Sarcina lutea, Escherichia coli, Salmonella typhi, Listeria monocytogenes, Helicobacter pylori, Streptococcus pyogenes, Salmonella* sp., *Mycobacterium tuberculosis, Mycobacterium avium, Klebsiella pneumoniae, Enterobacter aerogenes, Moraxella catarrhalis, Haemophilus influenzae, Neisseria meningitides, Enterococcus* spp., and *Bacillus cereus* [134, 135]. Bee propolis in combination with chlorhexidine possesses high antimicrobial activity against *Streptococcus mutans*. Propolis in combination with chlorhexidine can suppress the pathogenic potentials of a dental plaque by inhibiting the adherence and accumulation of cariogenic streptococci on the tooth surface.

Propolis has shown fungicidal effects on *Candida albicans; C. tropicalis; C. glabrata; C. famata; C.kefyr; C. pelliculosa; C. parapsilosis; C. guilliermondii; C. lusitaniae; C. stellatoidea; Cladosporium cladosporioides; C. sphaerospermum* [58]; *Pichia ohmeri; Trichosporon* sp. including *T. asahii, T. ovoides*, and *T. cutaneum; Geotrichum candidum; Saccharomyces cerevisiae; Rhodotorula* sp. [128]; and *Aspergillus niger* [58].The fungicidal effect was associated with the presence of flavonoids. Propolis microparticles from Brazilian propolis have shown their positive effect in the treatment of vulvovaginal candidiasis [128].

Antiprotozoal activity has been documented in the following diseases in humans and animals such as trichomoniasis (*Trichomonas vaginalis*), toxoplasmosis (*Toxoplasma gondii*), giardiasis

(*Giardia lamblia*), Chagas' disease (*Trypanosoma cruzi*), leishmaniasis (*Leishmania donovani*), and malaria (*P. falciparum, P. vivax, P. ovale, and P. malariae*) [128].

3.7. Side effects associated with the use of plant compound in wound management

The immune system is involved in skin allergies induced by plants. There are two different contact reactions mediated by the immune system in individuals sensitized to plants or plant products: immediate (type I) or delayed hypersensitivity contact reactions [136].

Aloe vera is frequently found in emollients, along with lanolin and parabens. It has been named a skin sensitizer because it may lead to a delayed hypersensitivity reaction [137].

Also curcumin is reported to have caused a few cases of contact allergy as a color agent in food or in disinfectants used prior to surgery [138].

The flower belonging to the family Compositae, including also *Calendula officinalis*, has induced many allergies in senior patients [139]. However, a study performed for a perfume made 100 % of *Calendula officinalis* did not influence the patch tests of patients allergic to the flower family Compositae [70]. On the other hand, specialists recommend to test additionally the creams containing *Calendula officinalis* because there have been patients that tested negative to Comp mix. (included in the standard patch test), but positive to the creams made with *Calendulaofficinalis* [139].

A few topical traditional Chinese medicaments have been involved in contact dermatitis: Saw Hong Choon skin ointment, Tjin Koo Lin, Tiger balm, Eagle brand oil, Green grass oil, White flower oil, Zhen Gu Shui, Tiger oil, and Wong Cheung Wah UI oil [140].

Regarding propolis allergic reactions, there have been reported with using red and green propolis. In green propolis, esters of aromatic acids, e.g., dimethyl allyl caffeic acid ester and flavonoids, e.g. tectochrysin, have been incriminated in producing contact dermatitis [126].

4. Conclusion

Many plants or plant-derived compounds with high levels of antioxidant properties and immunomodulatory and antimicrobial activity may have benefits in wound healing, being used for the design of bioactive wound dressings or topical formulations. However, the used methodology is inconsistent among different studies, and there is a lack of reports regarding the adverse effects of these plants, such as dermatitis. Therefore, in order to better exploit the huge reservoir of pharmacologically active plant-derived compounds and extracts, standardized methodology and clinical trials are necessary to give more concrete evidence supporting the use of traditional medicine in wound management.

Acknowledgements

The financial support of the research projects PN-III-P2-2.1-BG-2016-0369 and PN-III-P2-2.1-PTE-2016-0177 is gratefully acknowledged.

Author details

Mihaela Georgescu[1, 2, 3], Oana Marinas[2], Marcela Popa[3], Teodora Stan[2], Veronica Lazar[2, 3], Serban Vifor Bertesteanu[4, 5] and Mariana Carmen Chifiriuc[2,*]

* Address all correspondence to: carmen.chifiriuc@gmail.com; carmen_balotescu@yahoo.com

1 Dermatology Department, Central Universitary Emergency Military Hospital Dr Carol Davila, Bucharest, Romania

2 Microbiology Immunology Department, Faculty of Biology, University of Bucharest, Bucharest, Romania

3 Research Institute of the University of Bucharest (ICUB), Life, Environmental and Earth Sciences, Bucharest, Romania

4 University of Medicine and Pharmacy Carol Davila, University Emergency Hospital Bucharest, Bucharest, Romania

5 Head & Neck Surgery Clinic, Colţea Clinical Hospital, Bucharest, Romania

References

[1] Shai A, Maibach HI. Wound healing and ulcers of the skin, diagnosis and therapy—the practical approach. In : Marion Philipp, editor. Natural Course of Wound Repair Versus Impaired Healing in Chronic Skin Ulcers, Springer, 2005. 7–15

[2] Forsea D, Popescu R, Popescu CM. Dermatology and venerology compendium. Inferior leg ulcers. Technical Publishing House, 1996. p. 258–267

[3] Eming SA, Krieg T, Davidson JM. Inflammation in wound repair: molecular and cellular mechanisms. J Invest Dermatol.2007.127:514–25.

[4] Wolcott RD, Rhoads DD, Dowd SE. Biofilms and chronic wound inflammation. J Wound Care.2008. 17: 333–41

[5] Karapanagioti EG, Assimopoulou AN. Naturally occurring wound healing agents: An evidence-based review. Curr Med Chem. 2016 [Epub ahead of print]

[6] Hosseinkhani A, Falahatzadeh M, Raoofi E, Zarshenas MM. An evidence-based review on wound healing herbal remedies from reports of traditional Persian medicine. J Evid Based Complementary Altern Med. 2016 [Epub ahead of print]

[7] Thangapazham RL, Sharad S, Maheshwari RK. Phytochemicals in Wound Healing. Adv Wound Care (New Rochelle). 2016. 5(5):230–241.

[8] Kim TK, Shah S, Yang L. Controlling differentiation of adipose-derived stem cells using combinatorial graphene hybrid-pattern arrays. ACS Nano.2015. 9(4):3780–3790.

[9] Palombo EA. Traditional medicinal plant extracts and natural products with activity against oral bacteria: potential application in the prevention and treatment of oral diseases. Evid Based Complement Alternat Med. 2011;2011:680354

[10] Newman DJ, Cragg GM. Natural products as sources of new drugs over the last 25 years. J Nat Prod. 2007. 70(3):461–77

[11] Popa M, Hussien MD, Cirstea A, Grigore R, Lazar V, Bezirtzoglou E, Chifiriuc MC, Sakizlian M, Stavropoulou E, Bertesteanu S. Insights on metal based dental implants and their interaction with the surrounding tissues. Curr Top Med Chem. 2015. 15(16):1614–21

[12] Croteau R, Kutchan TM, Lewis NG. Natural products (secondary metabolites) in Buchanan B, Gruissem W, Jones R (Eds.), Biochemistry and molecular biology of plants. Rockville, MD: American Society of Plant Physiologists. 2000:1250–1318

[13] Istudor V. Phramacognosy, phytochemistry, phytotherapy. vol. II, Medical publishing house. Bucharest. 2001

[14] Bassole IHN, Juliani HR. Essential oils in combination and their antimicrobial properties, Molecules.2012. 17:3989-4006

[15] Nazzaro F, Fratianni F, De Martino L, Coppola R, De Feo V. Effect of essential oils on pathogenic bacteria. Pharmaceuticals. 2013. 6: 1451-1474

[16] Di Pasqua R, Betts G, Hoskins N, Edwards M, Ercolini D, Mauriello G. Membrane toxicity of antimicrobial compounds from essential oils. J. Agric. Food Chem.2007. 55: 4863–4870

[17] Nazzaro F, Fratianni F, Coppola R. Quorum sensing and phytochemicals. Int. J. Mol. Sci.2013. 14: 12607–12619

[18] Raut JS, Karuppayil SM. A status review on the medicinal properties of essential oils. Ind. Crops Prod. 2014. 62: 250–264

[19] Edris AE. Pharmaceutical and therapeutic potentials of essential oils and their individual volatile constituents: a review. Phytother. Res. Published online in Wiley InterScience (www.interscience.wiley.com) 2007. DOI: 10.1002/ptr.2072

[20] Bakkali F, Averbeck S, Averbeck D, Idaomar M. Biological effects of essential oils – a review. Food Chem. Toxicol. 2008. 46: 446–475

[21] Chaturvedi D. Opportunity, Challenge and Scope of Natural Products in Medicinal Chemistry, Sesquiterpene Lactones: Structural Diversity and their Biological Activities. Research Signpost, India. 2011. 37/661(2): 313–333

[22] Rodriguez-Amaya DB, Kimura M. Harvest Plus Handbook for Carotenoid Analysis. HarvestPlus Technical Monograph Series. 2004. 2: 2–7

[23] Cushnie TPT, Lamb AJ. Antimicrobial activity of flavonoids. J. Ethnopharmacol. 2005. 26: 343–356

[24] Borges A, Abreu AC, Malheiro J, Saavedra MJ, Simões M. Biofilm prevention and Control by Dietary Phytochemicals, Microbial Pathogens and Strategies for Combating them: Science, Technology and Education. Formatex Research Center; Editor: A. Méndez-Vilas; Microbiology Book Series – 2013 Edition. 2013. 1: 32–41

[25] Cueva C, Moreno-Arribas MV, Martin-Alvarez PJ, Bills G, Vicente MF, Basilio A, Rivas CL, Requena T, Rodriguez JM, Bartolome B. Antimicrobial activity of phenolic acids against commensal, probiotic and pathogenic bacteria. Res. Microbiol. 2010. 161: 372–382

[26] Mori A, Nishino C, Enoki N, Tawata S. Antibacterial activity and mode of action of plant flavonoids against *Proteus vulgaris* and *Staphylococcus aureus*. Phytochemistry. 1987. 26: 2231–2234

[27] Bernheim F. The effect of chloroform, phenols, alcohols and cyanogens iodide on the swelling of *Pseudomonas aeruginosa* in various salts. Microbios.1972. 5: 143

[28] Martin SA. Effects of extracellular pH and phenolic monomers on glucose uptake by Fibrobacter succinogenes S85. Ltr. Appl. Microbiol.1992. 15: 26–28

[29] Plaper A, Golob M, Hafner I, Oblak M, Solmajer T, Jerala R. Characterization of quercetin binding site on DNA gyrase. Biochem. Biophys. Res. Commun.2003. 306: 530–536

[30] Calixto JB, Otuki MF, Santos ARS. Anti-inflammatory compounds of plant origin. Part I. Action on arachidonic acid pathway, nitric oxide and nuclear factor kB(NF-kB). Planta Med.2003. 69: 973–983

[31] Chiang LC, Ng LT, Chang MY, Lin CC. Immunomodulatory activities of flavonoids, monoterpenoids, triterpenoids, iridoid glycosides and phenolic compounds of Plantago Species.Lanta Med. 2003. 69:600–604

[32] Kim HP, Son KH, Chang HW, Kang SS. Anti-inflammatory plant flavonoids and cellular action mechanisms. J. Pharmacol. Sci. 2004. 96: 229–245

[33] Yoon JH, Baek SJ. Molecular targets of dietary polyphenols with anti-inflammatory properties. Yonsei Med. J. 2005. 46: 585–596

[34] Chandrasekharan NV, Dai H, Roos KL, Evanson NK, Tomsik J, Elton TS, Simmons DL. COX-3, a cyclooxygenase-1 variant inhibited by acetaminophen and other analgesic/antipyretic drugs: cloning, structure, and expression. Proc Natl Acad Sci USA. 2002. 99: 13926–13931

[35] Needleman P, Isakson PC. The discovery and function of COX-2. J. Rheumatol. Suppl. 1997. 49: 6–8

[36] Middleton E Jr, Kandaswami C, Theoharides TC. The effects of plant flavonoids on mammalian cells: implications for inflammation, heart disease, and cancer. Pharmacol. Rev.2000. 52: 673–751

[37] Luceri C, Caderni G, Sanna A, Dolara P. Red wine and black tea polyphenols modulate the expression of cycloxygenase-2, inducible nitric oxide synthase and lutathione-related enzymes in azoxymethane-induced f344 rat colon tumors. J. Nutr.2002. 132: 1376–1379

[38] Miscalencu D, Caraene G, Mailat F, Nichita C. Efectele biologice benefice ale flavonoidelor. Ed. Universitatii din Bucuresti. 2008. pp. 21–24

[39] Laughton MJ, Evans PJ, Moroney MA, Hoult JR, Halliwell B. Inhibition of mammalian 5-lipoxygenase and cyclooxygenase by flavonoids and phenolic dietary additives. Relationship to antioxidant activity and to iron ion-reducing ability. Biochem. Pharmacol. 1991. 42: 1673–1681

[40] Kim HP, Mani I, Iversen L, Ziboh VA. Effects of naturallyoccurring flavonoids and biflavonoids on epidermal cyclooxygenase and lipoxygenase from guinea-pigs. Prostaglandins Leukot. Essent. Fatty Acids.1998. 58: 17–24

[41] Eo SH, Cho HS, Kim SJ. Resveratrol regulates type II collagen and COX-2 expression via the ERK, p38 and Akt signaling pathways in rabbit articular chondrocytes. Exp. Ther. Med. 2014. 7: 640–648

[42] Santangelo C, Vari R, Scazzocchio B, Di Benedetto R, Filesi C, Masella R. Polyphenols, intracellular signaling and inflammation. Ann Ist Super Sanità.2007. 43(4): 394–405

[43] Miles EA, Zoubouli P, Calder PC. Differential anti-inflammatory effects of phenolic compounds from extra virgin olive oil identified in human whole blood cultures. Nutrition. 2005. 21: 389–394

[44] Comalada M, Ballester I, Bailon E, Sierra S, Xaus J, Galvez J, de Medina FS, Zarzuelo A. Inhibition of pro-inflammatory markers in primary bone marrow-derived mouse macrophages by naturally occurring flavonoids: analysis of the structure-activity relationship. Biochem. Pharmacol.2006. 72: 1010–1021

[45] Sharma V, Mishra M, Ghosh S, Tewari R, Basu A, Seth P, Sen E. Modulation of interleukin-1beta mediated inflammatory response in human astrocytes by flavonoids: implications in neuroprotection. Brain Res. Bull. 2007. 73: 55–63

[46] Sato M, Miyazaki T, Kambe F, Maeda K, Seo H. Quercetin, a bioflavonoid, inhibits the induction of interleukin 8 and monocyte chemoattractant protein-1 expression by tumor necrosis factor-alpha in cultured human synovial cells. J. Rheumatol.1997. 24: 1680–1684

[47] Min YD, Choi CH, Bark H, Son HY, Park HH, Lee S, Park JW, Park EK, Shin HI, Kim SH. Quercetin inhibits expression of inflammatory cytokines through attenuation of NFkappaB and p38 MAPK in HMC-1 human mast cell line. Inflamm. Res.2007. 56: 210–215

[48] Kim IB, Kim DY, Lee SJ, Sun MJ, Lee MS, Li H, Cho JJ, Park CS. Inhibition of IL-8 production by green tea polyphenols in human nasal fibroblasts and a549 epithelial cells. Biol. Pharm. Bull. 2006. 29: 1120–1125

[49] Lyu SY, Park WB. Production of cytokine and NO by RAW 264.7 macrophages and PBMC in vitro incubation with flavonoids. Arch. Pharm. Res.2005. 28: 573–581

[50] Pan MH, Lai CS, Dushenkov S, Ho CT. Modulation of inflammatory genes by natural dietary bioactive compounds. J. Agric. Food Chem. 2009b. 57: 4467–4477

[51] Karin M, Ben-Neriah Y. Phosphorylation meets ubiquitination: the control of NF-[kappa] B activity. Annu. Rev. Immunol.2000. 18: 621–663

[52] Nam NH. Naturally occurring NF-kappaB inhibitors. Mini Rev. Med. Chem.2006. 6: 945–951

[53] Rahman I, Biswas SK, Kirkham PA. Regulation of inflammation and redox signaling by dietary polyphenols. Biochem. Pharmacol.2006. 72: 1439–1452

[54] Vanden Berghe W, Ndlovu MN, Hoya-Arias R, Dijsselbloem N, Gerlo S, Haegeman G. Keeping up NF-kappaB appearances: epigenetic control of immunity or inflammation-triggered epigenetics. Biochem. Pharmacol.2006. 72: 1114–1131

[55] Hayden MS, Ghosh S. Signaling to NF-kappaB. Genes Dev. 2004.18: 2195–2224

[56] Mackenzie GG, Carrasquedo F, Delfino JM, Keen CL, Fraga CG, Oteiza PI. Epicatechin, catechin, and dimeric procyanidins inhibit PMA-induced NF-kappaB activation at multiple steps in Jurkat T cells. FASEB J. 2004. 18: 167–169

[57] De Stefano D, Maiuri MC, Simeon V, Grassia G, Soscia A, Cinelli MP, Carnuccio R, Lycopene, quercetin and tyrosol prevent macrophage activation induced by gliadin and IFNgamma. Eur. J. Pharmacol.2007. 566:192–199

[58] Bankova V, Popova M, Trusheva B. Propolis volatile compounds: chemical diversity and biological activity: a review. Chem. Cent. J.2014:8:28

[59] Fokt H, Pereira A, Ferreira AM, Cunha A, Aguiar C. How does propolis prevent hive protection? The antimicrobial properties of propolis. Curr. Res. Tech. Educ. Top. Appl. Microbiol. Biotech. 2010:481–493

[60] Ugur A, Arslan T. An in vitro study on antimicrobial activity of propolis from Mugla province of Turkey. J. Med. Food. 2004. 7(1):90–4.

[61] Kujumgiev A, Tsvetkova I, Serkedjieva Y, Bankova V, Christov R, Popov S. Antibacterial, antifungal and antiviral activity of propolis of different geographic origin. J. Ethnopharmacol. 1999. 64(3):235–40.

[62] Stan Teodora. Investigation of biological effects and of mechanisms of action of Romanian propolis from different sources. PhD thesis. University of Bucharest, 2015

[63] Gebrehiwot M, Asres K, Bisrat D, Mazumder A, Lindemann P, Bucar F. Evaluation of the wound healing property of Commiphora guidottii Chiov. ex. Guid. BMC Complement Altern Med. 2015. 15:282

[64] Guimarães AL, Cunha EA, Matias FO, Garcia PG, Danopoulos P, Swikidisa R, Pinheiro VA, Nogueira RJ. Antimicrobial activity of Copaiba (*Copaifera officinalis*) and Pracaxi (*Pentaclethra macroloba*) oils against *Staphylococcus aureus*: importance in compounding for wound care. Int. J. Pharm. Compd. 2016. 20(1):58–62.

[65] Fahimi S, Abdollahi M, Mortazavi SA, Hajimehdipoor H, Abdolghaffari AH, Rezvanfar MA.Wound healing activity of a traditionally used poly herbal product in a burn wound model in rats. Iran Red Crescent Med. J. 2015. 17(9):e19960

[66] Léguillier T, Lecsö-Bornet M, Lémus C, Rousseau-Ralliard D, Lebouvier N, Hnawia E, Nour M, Aalbersberg W, Ghazi K, Raharivelomanana P, Rat P. The wound healing and antibacterial activity of five ethnomedical *Calophyllum inophyllum* oils: an alternative therapeutic strategy to treat infected wounds. PLoS One. 2015. 10(9):e0138602

[67] Bardaa S, Ben Halima N, Aloui F, Ben Mansour R, Jabeur H, Bouaziz M, Sahnoun Z. Oil from pumpkin (*Cucurbita pepo* L.) seeds: evaluation of its functional properties on wound healing in rats. Lipids Health Dis. 2016. 15:73

[68] Fan ZW, Pang YX, Wang K, Yu FL, Wang D, Yang Q, Ma QS, Li XT, Zou J, Zhang WQ,Wu LF. *Blumea balsamifera* oil for the acceleration of healing of burn injuries. Molecules. 2015. 20(9):17166–79

[69] http://ro.wikipedia.org/wiki/G%C4%83lbenele

[70] Paulsen E. Contact sensitization from Compositae-containing herbal remedies and cosmetics. Contact Dermatitis. 2002. 47:189–198

[71] Dinda M, Dasgupta U, Singh N, Bhattacharyya D, Karmakar P. PI3K-mediated proliferation of fibroblasts by *Calendula officinalis* tincture: implication in wound healing. Phytother. Res. 2015. 29: 607–616

[72] Arana L, Salado C, Vega S, Aizpurua-Olaizola O, Arada Ide L, Suarez T, Usobiaga A, Arrondo JL, Alonso A, Goñi FM, Alkorta I. Solid lipid nanoparticles for delivery of *Calendula officinalis* extract. Colloid Surf. B: Biointerfaces.2015. 135:18–26

[73] Butnariu M, Zepa Coradini C. Evaluation of biologically active compounds from *Calendula officinalis* flowers using spectrophotometry. Chem. Cent. J. 2012:6:35

[74] Herold A, Cremer L, Calugăru A, Tamaş V, Ionescu F, Manea S, Szegli G. Antioxidant properties of some hydroalcoholic plant extracts with antiinflammatory activity. Roum Arch. Microbiol. Immunol.. 2003. 62(3–4):217–27

[75] Parente LM, Lino Júnior R de S, Tresvenzol LM, Vinaud MC, de Paula JR, Paulo NM. Wound healing and anti-inflammatory effect in animal models of *Calendula officinalis* L. growing in Brazil. Evid. Based Complement. Alternat. Med. 2012. 2012: 375671

[76] Parente LM, Andrade MA, Brito LA, Moura VM, Miguel MP, Lino-Júnior RdeS, Tresvenzol LF, Paula JR, Paulo NM. Angiogenic activity of *Calendula officinalis* flowers L. in rats.Acta Cir. Bras..2011. 26(1):19–24

[77] Alonso G, Brandão C. Aloe vera for treating acute and chronic wounds. Sao Paulo Med J. 2014. 132(6):382

[78] Hashemi SA, Madani SA, Abediankenari S.The review on properties of aloe vera in healing of cutaneous wounds.Biomed. Res. Int. 2015. 2015:714216

[79] Maharjan H. Radha Nampoothiri P. Laxmipriya. Evaluation of biological properties and clinical effectiveness of aloe vera: a systematic review. J. Tradit. Complement Med.2015. 5(1): 21–26

[80] Benson KF, Newman RA, Jensen GS. Antioxidant, anti-inflammatory, anti-apoptotic, and skin regenerative properties of an Aloe vera-based extract of Nerium oleander leaves (NAE-8®). Clin. Cosmet. Investig. Dermatol. 2015. 8: 239–248

[81] Tummalapalli M, Berthet M, Verrier B, Deopura BL, Alam MS, Gupta B. Composite wound dressings of pectin and gelatin with aloe vera andcurcumin as bioactive agents. Int. J. Biol. Macromol. 2016. 82: 104–113

[82] Rahmani AH, Aldebasi YH, Srikar S, Khan AA, Aly SM. Aloe vera: potential candidate in health management via modulation of biological activities. Pharmacogn. Rev. 2015. 9(18): 120–126

[83] Sidgwick GP, McGeorge D, Bayat A. A comprehensive evidence-based review on the role of topicals and dressings in the management of skin scarring. Arch. Dermatol. Res.2015. 307(6): 461–477

[84] Thomas DR, Goode PS, LaMaster K, Tennyson T. Acemannan hydrogel dressing versus saline dressing for pressure ulcers. A randomized, controlled trial. Adv Wound Care. 1998. 11(6):273–6

[85] Silva SS, Caridade SG, Mano JF, Reis RL.Effect of crosslinking in chitosan/aloe vera-based membranes for biomedical applications. Carbohydr. Polym. 2013. 98(1):581–8

[86] Lin LX, Wang P, Wang YT, Huang Y, Jiang L, Wang XM. Aloe vera and Vitis vinifera improve wound healing in an in vivo rat burn wound model. Mol. Med. Rep. 2016. 13(2):1070–6

[87] Inpanya P, Faikrua A, Ounaroon A, Sittichokechaiwut A, Viyoch J. Effects of the blended fibroin/aloe gel film on wound healing in streptozotocin-induced diabetic rats. Biomed. Mater. 2012. 7(3):035008

[88] Panahi Y, Izadi M, Sayyadi N, Rezaee R, Jonaidi-Jafari N, Beiraghdar F, Zamani A, Sahebkar A. Comparative trial of Aloe vera/olive oil combination cream versus phenytoin cream in the treatment of chronic wounds. J. Wound Care. 2015. 24(10):459–60, 462–5.

[89] Mahmood K, Zia KM, Zuber M, Salman M, Anjum MN. Recent developments in curcumin and curcumin based polymeric materials for biomedical applications: A review. Int. J. Biol. Macromol. 2015. 81:877–90

[90] Naksuriya O, Okonogi S, Schiffelers RM, Hennink WE. Curcumin nanoformulations: a review of pharmaceutical properties and preclinical studies and clinical data related to cancer treatment. Biomaterials. 2014.35(10):3365–83

[91] Jardim KV, Joanitti GA, Azevedo RB, Parize AL. Physico-chemical characterization and cytotoxicity evaluation of curcumin loaded in chitosan/chondroitin sulfate nanoparticles. Mater. Sci. Eng. C Mater. Biol. Appl. 2015. 56:294–304

[92] Ranjbar-Mohammadi M, Bahrami SH. Electrospun curcumin loaded poly(-caprolactone)/gum tragacanthnanofibers for biomedical application. Int. J. Biol. Macromol. 2016. 84: 448–456

[93] Ghosh S, Banerjee S, Sil PC. The beneficial role of curcumin on inflammation, diabetes and neurodegenerative disease: a recent update. Food Chem. Toxicol.2015. 83:111–24

[94] Tyagi P, Singh M, Kumari H, Kumari A, Mukhopadhyay K. Bactericidal activity of curcumin I is associated with damaging of bacterial membrane. PLoS One. 2015. 10(3):e0121313.

[95] Izui S, Sekine S, Maeda K, Kuboniwa M, Takada A, Amano A, Nagata H. Antibacterial activity of curcumin against periodontopathic bacteria. J. Periodontol. 2016. 87(1):83–90

[96] Wang X, Ip M, Leung AW, Yang Z, Wang P, Zhang B, Ip S, Xu C.Sonodynamic action of curcumin on foodborne bacteria *Bacillus cereus* and *Escherichia coli*. Ultrasonics. 2015. 62:75–9.

[97] Mun SH, Joung DK, Kim YS, Kang OH, Kim SB, Seo YS, Kim YC, Lee DS, Shin DW, Kweon KT, Kwon DY.Synergistic antibacterial effect of curcumin against methicillin-resistant *Staphylococcus aureus*.Phytomedicine. 2013. 20(8–9):714–8

[98] Bhaskar Rao A, Prasad E, Deepthi SS, Haritha V, Ramakrishna S, Madhusudan K, Surekha MV, Venkata Rao YS. Wound healing: a new perspective on glucosylated tetrahydrocurcumin. Drug Des. Dev. Ther. 2015. 9:3579–88

[99] Bhagavathula N, Warner RL, DaSilva M, McClintock SD, Barron A, Aslam MN, Johnson KJ, Varani J. A combination of curcumin and ginger extract improves abrasion wound healing in corticosteroid-impaired hairless rat skin. Wound Repair Regen.2009. 17(3):360–6

[100] Topman G, Lin FH, Gefen A. The natural medications for wound healing—Curcumin, Aloe-Vera and Ginger—do not induce a significant effect on the migration kinematics of cultured fibroblasts. J. Biomech..2013. 46(1):170–4

[101] Alerico GC, Beckenkamp A, Vignoli-Silva M, Buffon A, von Poser GL. Proliferative effect of plants used for wound healing in Rio Grande do Sul state, Brazil. J. Ethnopharmacol. 2015. 176:305–10

[102] Dos Santos Gramma LS, Marques FM, Vittorazzi C, de Andrade TA, Frade MA, de Andrade TU, Endringer DC, Scherer R, Fronza M. Struthanthus vulgaris ointment prevents an over expression of inflammatory response and accelerates the cutaneous wound healing. J. Ethnopharmacol. 2016. 190:319–327.

[103] Geller FC, Teixeira MR, Pereira AB, Dourado LP, Souza DG, Braga FC, Simões CM. Evaluation of the wound healing properties of Hancornia speciosa leaves. Phytother. Res. 2015. 29(12):1887–93

[104] de Campos EP, Trombini LN, Rodrigues R, Portella DL, Werner AC, Ferraz MC, de Oliveira RV, Cogo JC, Oshima-Franco Y, Aranha N, Gerenutti M. Healing activity of Casearia sylvestris Sw. in second-degree scald burns in rodents. BMC Res Notes. 2015. 8:269

[105] Kıyan S, Uyanıkgil Y, Altuncı YA, Çavuşoğlu T, Çetin Uyanıkgil EÖ, Karabey F. Investigation of acute effects of Hypericum perforatum (St. John's Wort-Kantaron) treatment in experimental thermal burns and comparison with silver sulfadiazine treatment. Ulus Travma Acil Cerrahi Derg. 2015. 21(5):323–36

[106] Eruygur N, Yılmaz G, Kutsal O, Yücel G, Üstün O. Bioassay-guided isolation of wound healing active compounds from Echium species growing in Turkey. J. Ethnopharmacol. 2016. 185:370–6

[107] Agar OT, Dikmen M, Ozturk N, Yilmaz MA, Temel H, Turkmenoglu FP. Comparative studies on phenolic composition, antioxidant, wound healing and cytotoxic activities of selected Achillea L. species growing in Turkey. Molecules. 2015. 20(10):17976–8000

[108] Agyare C, Boakye YD, Bekoe EO, Hensel A, Dapaah SO, Appiah T. Review: African medicinal plants with wound healing properties. J. Ethnopharmacol. 2016. 177:85–100

[109] Mulisa E, Asres K, Engidawork E. Evaluation of wound healing and anti-inflammatory activity of the rhizomes of Rumex abyssinicus J. (Polygonaceae) in mice. BMC Complement Altern Med. 2015. 15:341.

[110] Spiegler V, Sendker J, Petereit F, Liebau E, Hensel A. Bioassay-guided fractionation of a leaf extract from *Combretum mucronatum* with anthelmintic activity: oligomeric procyanidins as the active principle. Molecules. 2015. 20(8):14810–32.

[111] Imran H, Ahmad M, Rahman A, Yaqeen Z, Sohail T, Fatima N, Iqbal W, Yaqeen SS. Evaluation of wound healing effects between *Salvadora persica* ointment and Solcoseryl jelly in animal model. Pak. J. Pharm. Sci. 2015. 28(5):1777–80.

[112] Tsala DE, Nga N, Thiery BN, Bienvenue MT, Theophile D. Evaluation of the antioxidant activity and the healing action of the ethanol extract of *Calotropis procera* bark against surgical wounds. J. Intercult. Ethnopharmacol. 2015. 4(1):64–9.

[113] Patil RA, Makwana AB. Anti-hyperbilirubinemic and wound healing activity of aqueous extract of *Calotropis procera* leaves in Wistar rats. Indian J. Pharmacol. 2015. 47(4):398–402

[114] Gothai S, Arulselvan P, Tan WS, Fakurazi S. Wound healing properties of ethyl acetate fraction of *Moringa oleifera* in normal human dermal fibroblasts. J. Intercult. Ethnopharmacol. 2016. 5(1):1–6

[115] Seo SH, Lee SH, Cha PH, Kim MY, Min do S, Choi KY. *Polygonum aviculare* L. and its active compounds, quercitrin hydrate, caffeic acid, and rutin, activate the Wnt/β-catenin pathway and induce cutaneous wound healing. Phytother. Res. 2016. 30(5):848–54.

[116] Jácomo AC, de Andrade Velozo K, Lotti RG, Neves LM, de Gaspari de Gaspi FO, Esquisatto MA, do Amaral ME, Mendonça FA, dos Santos GM. Activity of Porophyllum ruderale leaf extract and 670-nm InGaP laser during burns repair in rats. BMC Complement Altern. Med. 2015. 15:274

[117] Saenthaweesuk S, Jitvaropas R, Somparn N, Thuppia A.An investigation of antimicrobial and wound healing potential of *Allium ascalonicum* Linn. J. Med. Assoc. Thai. 2015;98 Suppl 2:S22–7.

[118] Lee K, Lee B, Lee MH, Kim B, Chinannai KS, Ham I, Choi HY. Effect of Ampelopsis Radix on wound healing in scalded rats. BMC Complement Altern. Med. 2015. 15:213

[119] George BP, Parimelazhagan T, Kumar YT, Sajeesh T. Antitumor and wound healing properties of *Rubus ellipticus* Smith. J. Acupunct. Meridian Stud. 2015. 8(3):134–41

[120] Von Atzingen DA, Mendonça AR, Mesquita Filho M, Alvarenga VA, Assis VA, Penazzo AE, Muzetti JH, Rezende TS. Repair of surgical wounds in rats using a 10% unripe Musa sapientum peel gel. Acta Cir. Bras.. 2015. 30(9):586–92

[121] Mohamed Amin Z, Koh SP, Yeap SK, Abdul Hamid NS, Tan CP, Long K. Efficacy study of broken rice maltodextrin in in vitro wound healing assay. Biomed. Res. Int. 2015. 2015:687694

[122] Rushdi AI, Adgaba N, Bayaqoob NI, Al-Khazim A, Simoneit BI, El-Mubarak AH, Al-Mutlaq KF. Characteristics and chemical compositions of propolis from Ethiopia. Springerplus. 2014. 3:253

[123] Silva-Carvalho R, Baltazar F, Almeida-Aguiar C. Propolis: a complex natural product with a plethora of biological activities that can be explored for drug development. Evid. Based Complement Alternat. Med. 2015. 2015:206439

[124] Henshaw FR, Bolton T, Nube V, Hood A, Veldhoen D, Pfrunder L, McKew GL, Macleod C, McLennan SV, Twigg SM. Topical application of the bee hive protectant propolis is well tolerated and improves human diabetic foot ulcer healing in a prospective feasibility study. J. Diabetes Complic. 2014. 28(6):850–7

[125] de Moura SA, Negri G, Salatino A, Lima LD, Dourado LP, Mendes JB, Andrade SP, Ferreira MA, Cara DC. Aqueous extract of brazilian green propolis: primary components, evaluation of inflammation and wound healing by using subcutaneous implanted sponges. Evid. Based Complement Alternat. Med. 2011. 2011:748283

[126] de Almeida EB, Cordeiro Cardoso J, Karla de Lima A, de Oliveira NL, de Pontes-Filho NT, Oliveira Lima S, Leal Souza IC, de Albuquerque-Júnior RL. The incorporation of Brazilian propolis into collagen–based dressing films improves dermal burn healing. J. Ethnopharmacol. 2013. 147(2):419–25

[127] Tolba MF, Omar HA, Azab SS, Khalifa AE, Abdel-Naim AB, Abdel-Rahman SZ. Caffeic acid phenethyl ester: A review of its antioxidant activity, protective effects against ischemia-reperfusion injury and drug adverse reactions. Crit. Rev. Food Sci. Nutr. 2014 3:0. [Epub ahead of print]

[128] Wagh VD. Propolis: a wonder bees product and its pharmacological potentials. Adv. Pharmacol. Sci. 2013. 2013:308249

[129] Hozzein WN, Badr G, Al Ghamdi AA, Sayed A, Al-Waili NS, Garraud O. Topical application of propolis enhances cutaneous wound healing by promoting TGF-beta/Smad-mediated collagen production in a streptozotocin-induced type I diabetic mouse model. Cell Physiol. Biochem. 2015. 37(3):940–54

[130] Lima LD, Andrade SP, Campos PP, Barcelos LS, Soriani FM, Moura SA, Ferreira MA. Brazilian green propolis modulates inflammation, angiogenesis and fibrogenesis in intraperitoneal implant in mice. BMC Complement Altern. Med. 2014. 14:177

[131] Takzaree N, Hadjiakhondi A, Hassanzadeh G, Rouini MR, Manayi A. Synergistic effect of honey and propolis on cutaneous wound healing in rats. Acta Med. Iran. 2016. 54(4):233–9.

[132] Oryan A, Alemzadeh E, Moshiri A. Biological properties and therapeutic activities of honey in wound healing: A narrative review and meta-analysis. J. Tissue Viab. 2016. 25(2):98–118.

[133] Barud Hda S, de Araújo Júnior AM, Saska S, Mestieri LB, Campos JA, de Freitas RM, Ferreira NU, Nascimento AP, Miguel FG, Vaz MM, Barizon EA, Marquele-Oliveira F, Gaspar AM, Ribeiro SJ, Berretta AA. Antimicrobial Brazilian Propolis (EPP-AF) containing biocellulose membranes as promising biomaterial for skin wound healing. Evid. Based Complement Alternat. Med. 2013. 2013:703024

[134] Kurek-Górecka A, Rzepecka-Stojko A, Górecki M, Stojko J, Sosada M, Swierczek-Zieba G. Structure and antioxidant activity of polyphenols derived from propolis. Molecules. 2013. 19(1):78–101

[135] De Vecchi E, Drago L. Propolis' antimicrobial activity: what's new? Infez Med. 2007. 15(1):7–15.

[136] Mantle D, Gok MA, Lennard TW. Adverse and beneficial effects of plant extracts on skin and skin disorders. Adverse Drug React. Toxicol. Rev.2001. 20(2):89–103

[137] White-Chu EF, Reddy M.Dry skin in the elderly: complexities of a common problem. Clin. Dermatol. 2011. 29(1):37–42

[138] Rastogi SC, Johansen JD. Colourants in transferable picture tattoos for the skin. Contact Dermatitis. 2005. 53(4):207–10

[139] Reider N, Komericki P, Hausen BM, Fritsch P, Aberer W. The seamy side of natural medicines: contact sensitization to arnica (*Arnica montana* L.) and marigold (*Calendula officinalis* L.). Contact Dermatitis. 2001.45(5):269–72

[140] Lim KS, Tang MB, Goon AT, Leow YH. Contact sensitization in patients with chronic venous leg ulcers in Singapore. Contact Dermatitis. 2007. 56(2):94–8

Section 2

Development of Conventional Methodology and Quality of Life

Chapter 5

Nursing Interventions in Prevention and Healing of Leg Ulcers: Systematic Review of the Literature

César Fonseca , Manuel Lopes , Ana Ramos ,
Vitor Santos , Antonio Esquinas and Pedro Parreira

Additional information is available at the end of the chapter

http://dx.doi.org/10.5772/65719

Abstract

Aim: The purpose of this study was to define nursing interventions for patients with venous, arterial or mixed leg ulcers.

Methodology: A survey was conducted in EBSCO (CINAHL Plus with Full Text, MEDLINE with Full Text), MedicLatina, Academic Search Complete, with full text articles, published between 2008/01/01 and 2015/01/31, with the following keywords: [(MM "leg ulcer") OR (wound care) OR (wound healing)] AND [(nursing) OR (nursing assessment) OR (nursing intervention)].

Results: The different leg ulcer etiologies require different therapeutic approach to prevention and treatment. Predictive factors were identified associated with healing: patient-centred care, interpersonal relationship, pain control, control of the exudate, education for health self-management, self-care, therapeutic compliance, implementation of guidelines, auditing and feedback on the practices.

Conclusion: Evidence-based practice helps to improve efficiency, safety and quality of nursing care directed to people with leg ulcers or at risk of developing this type of wounds.

Keywords: nursing interventions, leg ulcer, prevention and treatment

1. Introduction

Currently, the needs of healthcare clients are increasingly demanding and complex, as a result of the increase in average life expectancy [1, 2], and the resulting prevalence of chronic illnesses, such as leg ulcers. The possibility of ulceration increases with age, due to which an exponential increase in its incidence and prevalence is expected [3]. Leg ulcers can be defined as ulceration below the knee on any part of the leg [4], including the foot, and is classified as a chronic wound, that is, a wound that remains stuck in any of the phases of the healing process for a period of 6 weeks or more, or that requires a structured intervention of nursing care [5, 6]. There are several known leg ulcer aetiologies, among which those of venous origin are the most common, at 70% of the cases, followed by those that are arterial in origin, at 10–20% of the cases, and those of a mixed aetiology, at 10–15% of the cases [7]. The main causes of the appearance of leg ulcers are chronic venous hypertension, arterial disease or a combination of the two [5, 6]. The less-frequent causes are neuropathy, infection, vasculitis, neoplasia, blood and metabolic disorders, or lymphedema and disorders that are iatrogenic in origin [5, 6]. The relevance of this problem is supported by statistics, in which 1.5–3 in every 1000 individuals have leg ulcers, with increased prevalence at higher ages, leading to 20 for every 1000 individuals aged more than 80 years [2, 8]. The literature mentions that leg ulcers are interpreted as "a forever healing experience" [9, 10], associated with the fact that 50% of the time, primary healthcare nurses are involved in treating leg ulcers, with the presence of pain in 49–90% of cases, where 50% of venous ulcers heal after 4 months, 20% of venous ulcers heal in between 4 months and 1 year, 20% require a period greater than 2 years to heal, 8% remain unhealed even after 8 years and 69–26% recur in the first year [9].

The repercussions of leg ulcers also have an effect on healthcare expenditure, wherein 1–2% of the total health budget in Western countries [11], of which Portugal is part, is directed to this type of chronic wound [4, 12, 13]. In European countries, an economical investment of approximately 6.5 million Euros/year is estimated in the treatment of leg ulcers [14]. Its impact interferes significantly with human lifestyles, affecting the performance of day-to-day activities, quality of life, functional capacity and self-esteem, leading to workplace absenteeism, financial problems, isolation, sleep disorders and the development of mental illness [15, 16].

Hence, a systematisation is proposed of nursing interventions aimed at persons with venous, arterial or mixed leg ulcers.

2. Methodology

Carried out research in the EBSCO search engine: CINAHL Plus with Full Text, MEDLINE with Full Text, MedicLatina, Academic Search Complete, sought full-text articles, published between 2008/01/01 and 2015/01/31, with the following keywords: [(MM "leg ulcer") OR (wound care) OR (wound healing)] AND [(nursing) OR (nursing assessment) OR (nursing intervention)], filtered through initial question in PI[C]O format. As a starting point in the systematic review of the literature, the following question was formulated in PI[C]O [16] format: "In relation to persons with venous, arterial and mixed leg ulcers (Population), what are the nursing interventions (Intervention) that can influence healing (Outcomes)?" The EBSCO search engine was queried, with access to two databases: CINAHL Plus with Full Text,

MEDLINE with Full Text, MedicLatina, Academic Search Complete, sought full text articles, published between 2008/01/01 and 2015/01/31, with the following keywords: [(MM "leg ulcer") OR (wound care) OR (wound healing)] AND [(nursing) OR (nursing assessment) OR (nursing intervention)].

The process for searching and selecting material for analysis is explained in **Table 1**.

	Protocol
↓	**Identification:**
	• No. of cases identified: CINAHL -310 • No. of cases identified: MEDLINE – 433 • No. of cases identified: MedicLatina - 31 • No. of cases identified: Academic Search Complete - 24
	Screening:
	• No. of duplicated cases that were removed – 384 • No. of cases selected – 414
	Inclusion Criteria (complete reading):
	• No. of full text articles with inclusion criteria - 11 • No. of full text articles without inclusion criteria - 403
	Articles Included (levels of evidence[16]): Level I – 2; Level II – 1; Level IV – 3; Level V – 4; Level VI – 1

Table 1. Process for searching and selection for the systematic review of the literature.

3. Results

In order to make the methodology used easy to understand and transparent, the list of 12 articles selected is explained (**Table 2**) for the body of analysis, which formed the basis for the preparation of the discussion and the corresponding conclusions, having been subjected to classification by levels of evidence.

Level of evidence/ articles	**Method**	**Participants**	**Interventions**	**Results**
Level of evidence— V [17]	Systematic review of the literature	Review of three guidelines	Critical review of the guidelines in order to	Recommendations are prepared on how to assess leg ulcers, as well as

Level of evidence/ articles	Method	Participants	Interventions	Results
		(Medline and Cochrane)	prepare a set of recommendations	how to treat the different aetiologies: venous, arterial and mixed
Level of evidence— V [8]	Systematic review of the literature	31 articles relating to people with venous and/or mixed leg ulcers	The articles were analysed in order to be able to perceive failure To comply with the treatment	Pain, discomfort and different lifestyles are some of the reasons why leg ulcer patients did not comply with the treatment. Healthcare professionals must focus on problems reported by the patients in order to be able to help them overcome these problems and to motivate them to take the treatment
Level of evidence— V [14]	Systematic review of the literature	Publications on social support and persons with leg ulcers	Several studies are compared in order to establish a relationship between the effect of social support on the healing of venous leg ulcers as well as on recurrence	Social support is important for persons with venous leg ulcers, as this support is necessary during as well as after the wound is healed, in order to prevent recurrence
Level of evidence— V [18]	RCT	All the people with leg ulcers in the region of Skaraborg (Sweden).	Identification of people with leg ulcers, their aetiology, prevalence and ongoing treatment	It was observed that venous leg ulcers continue to be the most prevalent, followed by arterial leg ulcers. In general, there is a reduction in prevalence in relation to previous studies
Level of evidence— I [19]	Systematic review of the literature	325 database articles (Cinahl, Medline and Cochrane)	Critical review of the articles found in order to prepare a set of recommendations	Recommendations are prepared on how to assess and intervene among patients with arterial leg ulcers, on the following points: debridement, dressing selection, infection control, nutrition, pain control
Level of evidence— I [20]	Systematic review of the literature	180 database articles (Medline and Cochrane)	Critical review of the articles found in order to prepare a set of recommendations	Recommendations are prepared on how to assess, prevent and treat people with venous leg ulcers
Level of evidence— IV [6]	Retrospective study	Eight people with mixed leg ulcers treated by two specialist nurses	Identify the role of the specialist nurse in controlling ulceration	The ulcers heal in between 6 and 30 weeks after the first application of an inelastic bandage system. This intervention was well tolerated by all

http://dx.doi.org/10.5772/65719

Level of evidence/ articles	Method	Participants	Interventions	Results
				the patients, and no adverse effects were recorded
Level of evidence—IV [12]	Prospective study	Five persons with leg ulcers, with assistance at home and over the telephone, for 12 weeks	Identify the strategies in the promotion of therapeutic compliance	Individualisation of information, training/instruction increases therapeutic compliance
Level of evidence—V [13]	Systematic review of the literature	Five articles resulting from searches on MEDLINE, British Nursing Index and Cumulative Index to Nursing and Allied Health Literature (CINAHL)	Control the level of exudate in leg ulcers	Proper control of the amount of exudate minimises the impact on quality of life, damage to the wound bed, on the perilesional skin, reduces the risk of infection, days required for healing of the wound and health expenditure
Level of evidence—VI [3]	Case study	A person with a venous leg ulcer	Analyse the influence of self-care on leg ulcer healing	The capacity for self-care stimulated by the patient's empowerment reduces the need for seeking health care
Level of evidence—IV [21]	Case study—control	11 persons with pressure ulcers and 20 with leg ulcers, in primary care	Verify the advantages of the use of absorbent dressings in controlling the exudate of venous ulcers	The control of exudate promotes healing of chronic wounds, control of pain and negative psychosocial effects associated with the smell and change of dressings

Table 2. Body of analysis.

4. Discussion of the data

The evaluation of the awareness, expectations, quality of social support, need for information enables the adaptation of education, training and instruction on healthy lifestyles, wound care, physical exercise and elevation of lower limbs in venous aetiology. The patient, on feeling involved, with the use of an easy-to-understand language, increases his or her motivation, self-efficacy and capacity for self-care [12].

The creation of spaces (Leg Clubs) has proved to be a fundamental strategy in therapeutic compliance [10], where nurses with specific training in the area of leg ulcers promote social interaction between patients with the same type of ulcer, evaluate the support required by each individual, provide training aimed at self-care and case management, provide the corresponding treatment and constant monitoring [4–9]. The result of the implementation of this project was the reduction in pain intensity, significant progress in healing and an increase in quality of life, specifically at the workplace, in moods, in mobility, sleep patterns and other aspects [10]. The positive effect of this model is also reflected at the social level [9], given that more extended social contact with people who have or have had the same problem, reduces social isolation and provides effective coping mechanisms for dealing with the crisis situation - the illness [3, 4, 16].

<table>
<tr><th>Venous ulcer</th><th>Arterial ulcer</th><th>Mixed ulcer</th></tr>
<tr>
<td rowspan="2">• Apply compressive therapy if the Ankle-Brachial Index (ABI) is greater than 0.8
• Select the type of compression to be used: multi-layer compression system below the knee (general treatment); reduced compression system (in case the patient does not tolerate higher compressions); compression stockings (after the ulcer's healing); intermittent compression system (can be used in isolation or together with another compression system, in order to increase venous return)
• Select the compressive therapy material to be used: elastic bandages (long-stretch), considered more effective; non-elastic bandages (short-stretch), which cause less discomfort/pain; multi-layer elastic bandage systems (two, three or four layers); elastic stockings; multi-layered elastic stockings; zinc-impregnated bandage (Unna Boot) together with elastic bandages
• Apply compression stockings with customised measurement, if the ulcer has healed
• Refer for vascular surgery in the following situations: no reduction in the size of the ulcer after 30 days of treatment; ulcer present for more than 6 months; intolerance to compressive therapy; ineffectiveness in pain control; frequent recurrence</td>
<td>• Assess the lower limbs, frequently, in relation to: functional capacity; colouring, temperature; capillary reperfusion; sensitivity; presence of dorsalis pedis, posterior tibial pulse; signs of neuropathy
• Perform cleaning of the wound with non-cytotoxic products
• Do not debride dry and stable necrotic tissue without proper assessment of the perfusion through vascular surgery, not applying any moisture retaining bandage material
• Debride the necrotic tissue, based on a multi-professional decision, using autolytic and enzymatic debridement</td>
<td>• Apply reduced compression (between 23 and 30 mmHg) in the presence of oedema
• Refer for vascular surgery, if there is no healing development and ABI is lower than 0.5</td>
</tr>
<tr>
<td colspan="2">• Provide training in the following structural areas: control of associated pathologies; giving up smoking and drinking; encouraging the ingestion of food rich in vitamin B6 (increases HDL-C and reduces triglycerides), such as potato, banana, chicken breast, sunflower seeds, salmon, tuna, avocado, and others; prevention of chemical, thermal or mechanical trauma on the lower limbs; skin care; use of sui footwear and non-compressive stockings
• Institute a regular physical exercise programme, for patients with intermittent claudication, based on 30–60-min walks (3 days a week at least), wherein the patient may stop and rest in case of pain
• Refer to vascular surgery if: ABI is lower than 0.8; signs and symptoms of infection; continued pain at rest, even with the limb dropped; absence of both, pedis and posterior tibial pulses
• If ABI is lower than 0.5, refer urgently for observation by vascular surgery</td>
</tr>
</table>

Table 3. Nursing interventions in venous, arterial and mixed leg ulcers.

http://dx.doi.org/10.5772/65719

On initial assessment, it is crucial to cover the history of health: associated co-morbidities, habitual therapy, psycho-emotional state, influence of odour on social life, nutritional state, presence and intensity of pain and individual treatment preference. In evaluating the amount of exudate, it is recommended to document the saturation of the absorbent dressing and support/compression bandage, instead of rating it as minimum (+), moderate (++) and high (+++), in order to increase the record's objectivity. If the perilesional skin is macerated, this indicates that the dressings must be applied more frequently, or that the selected material is not the most suited for controlling the exudate. In leg ulcers subjected to compression therapy, in venous aetiology, dressings that allow for evaporation of the exudate through their semi-permeable covering cease to be effective. In light of the above, the use of hydrofibre and alginates is recommended. The application of negative pressure on the wound bed and the use of protective sprays/creams on the surrounding area are measures to be considered in the case of ulcers with hard-to-control exudate [13, 14].

The application of compression bandages is considered an essential element in the treatment of venous leg ulcers. The effect of compression on mixed leg ulcers can be beneficial in reducing local oedema, in improving microcirculation, contributing to improving arterial flow and improving venous as well as lymphatic drainage. Still, the application of compression on legs with mixed aetiology requires strong additional care, as it is generally contraindicated for the reduction of arterial flow, causing greater tissue damage, as shown in study [6], with the use of inelastic bandage. The number of layers to be applied is normally decided based on the malleolar circumference, based on the manufacturer's instructions (one layer is applied when the malleolar circumference is ≤25 cm, and two layers when it is >25 cm). However, in mixed aetiology, it is recommended to start the treatment with only one layer, for less-elevated compression levels. The interventions provided by specialist nurses when dealing with chronic wounds increase gains in health, due to their expertise in using tools for assessing compressive therapy: Doppler ultrasound and ankle-brachial index (ABI).

Concerning nursing interventions in the prevention and treatment of venous, arterial or mixed leg ulcers, it is fundamental to know the patient's clinical history (personal background, chronic pathologies, current state of the client) and the history of the ulcer (source, time, treatments performed) [6, 12, 14–16, 18, 22–24]. On meticulously evaluating the characteristics of the wound (size, depth, exudate, wound bed, type of tissues, perilesional skin, pain) [4, 18], the decision must be made in partnership with the client (**Table 3**) in order to establish common goals [15, 17–21].

Thus, the treatment must involve pain prevention [10], preparation of the wound bed [6–9], wound cleaning [14–16], management of products to be applied to the bed and perilesional skin [7], joint selection of the type of material for application of compressive treatment and preparation of a physical exercise plan [8, 14–16, 18, 22], continuous client empowerment [17], referral to specialities in case of allergic reactions [13], need for supplementary therapies and/or non-effective treatments carried out in which the ulcer/state of the client deteriorates.

5. Conclusions and implications for the practice of nursing

The presence of social support was the aspect most mentioned by the people as essential in their process of adaptation, whether provided by significant persons, or through contact with people in similar situations (self-help groups) or by the nurse. The education for health self-management was considered of utmost importance in controlling other associated chronic illnesses, in the reduction of other existing risk factors and for creating physiological conditions that favoured better healing. The monitoring of the ulcer's characteristics, physical activity, nutritional diet, favoured healing and improved the perceived quality of life. Continuous and up-to-date training of nurses providing care to leg ulcer patients emerged as another aspect positively associated with the effectiveness and excellence of the interventions carried out.

An approach centred on the patient and on pain control, mainly when the therapeutic plan involves compression on the wound bed, is key determinants in increasing participation and involvement in the therapeutic plan.

Conflicts of interest

The author declares no conflict of interest.

Author details

César Fonseca[1*], Manuel Lopes[1], Ana Ramos[2], Vitor Santos[1], Antonio Esquinas[3] and Pedro Parreira[4]

*Address all correspondence to: cesar.j.fonseca@gmail.com

1 University of Évora, Évora, Portugal

2 Hospital Middle Tejo Center, Tomar, Portugal

3 Intensive Care Unit, Hospital Morales Meseguer, Murcia, Spain

4 Coimbra Nursing School, Coimbra, Portugal

References

[1] Instituto Nacional de Estatística. *Projecções de População Residente em Portugal 2008–2060*. Instituto Nacional de Estatistica – Ministério da Saúde.. Portugal. Lisboa. 2014.

[2] Van Hecke A, Grypdonck M, Defloor T. A review of why patients with leg ulcers do not adhere to treatment. *Journal of Clinical Nursing* [serial on the Internet]. (2009, Feb),

[cited January 4, 2015]; 18(3): 337–349. http://search.ebscohost.com/login.aspx?direct=true&db=rzh&AN=105629598&site=ehost-live

[3] Yarwood-Ross L, Haigh C. Managing a venous leg ulcer in the 21st century, by improving self-care. *British Journal Of Community Nursing* [serial online]. October 2012;17(10):460–465. http://search.ebscohost.com/login.aspx?direct=true&db=rzh&AN=108112049&site=ehost-live

[4] Brown A. Does social support impact on venous ulcer healing or recurrence?. *British Journal of Community Nursing* [serial on the Internet]. (2008, Mar 2), [cited January 4, 2015]; 13(3): S6. http://search.ebscohost.com/login.aspx?direct=true&db=rzh&AN=105909037&site=ehost-live

[5] Werchek S. Diagnosis and treatment of venous leg ulcers. *The Nurse Practitioner* [serial on the Internet]. (2010, Dec), [cited January 4, 2015]; 35(12): 46–53. http://search.ebscohost.com/login.aspx?direct=true&db=rzh&AN=104972282&site=ehost-live

[6] Neill K, Turnbull K. Use of specialist knowledge and experience to manage patients with mixed aetiology leg ulcers. *Journal Of Wound Care* [serial online]. April 2012;21(4):168–174. http://search.ebscohost.com/login.aspx?direct=true&db=rzh&AN=104422923&site=ehost-live

[7] Vowden P. Leg ulcers: assessment and management. *Independent Nurse* [serial on the Internet]. (2010, Nov 22), [cited January 4, 2015]; 12(3): 30–33. http://search.ebscohost.com/login.aspx?direct=true&db=rzh&AN=104956673&site=ehost-live

[8] Hecke A, Grypdonck M, Defloor T. Interventions to enhance patient compliance with leg ulcer treatment: a review of the literature. *Journal of Clinical Nursing* [serial on the Internet]. (2008, Jan), [cited January 4, 2015]; 17(1): 29–39. http://search.ebscohost.com/login.aspx?direct=true&db=rzh&AN=106013847&site=ehost-live

[9] Chamanga E. How can community nurses improve quality of life for patients with leg ulcers?. *Nursing Times* [serial online]. March 16, 2010;106(10):15–17. http://search.ebscohost.com/login.aspx?direct=true&db=mnh&AN=20426295&site=ehost-live

[10] Ebbeskog B, Emami A. Older patients' experience of dressing changes on venous leg ulcers: more than just a docile patient. *Journal of Clinical Nursing* [serial on the Internet]. (2005, Nov), [cited January 4, 2015]; 14(10): 1223–1231. http://search.ebscohost.com/login.aspx?direct=true&db=rzh&AN=106385326&site=ehost-live

[11] EUROSTAT. Population projections 2008–2060: from 2015, deaths projected to outnumber births in the EU27. S.1: Eurostat Press Office; Lanzieri: Eurostat News. 2008:1–4. Available from: http://ec.europa.eu/eurostat

[12] Van Hecke A, Beeckman D, Grypdonck M, Meuleneire F, Hermie L, Verhaeghe S. Knowledge Deficits and Information-Seeking Behavior in Leg Ulcer Patients: An Exploratory Qualitative Study. *Journal Of Wound, Ostomy & Continence Nursing*

[serial online]. July 2013;40(4):381–387. http://search.ebscohost.com/login.aspx?direct=true&db=rzh&AN=107958718&site=ehost-live

[13] Menon J. Managing exudate associated with venous leg ulceration. *British Journal Of Community Nursing* [serial online]. June 2, 2012; 25(4):S6–s16. http://search.ebscohost.com/login.aspx?direct=true&db=mnh&AN=22875033&site=ehost-live

[14] Martin F. Educational challenges and requirements for managing leg ulcers in the communi. *British Journal Of Community Nursing* [serial online]. June 2, 2014; 12(2):S32–6. http://search.ebscohost.com/login.aspx?direct=true&db=rzh&AN=103960614&site=ehost-live

[15] Edwards H, Courtney M, Finlayson K, Lindsay E, Lewis C, Chang A, et al. Chronic venous leg ulcers: effect of a community nursing intervention on pain and healing. *Nursing Standard* [serial on the Internet]. (2005, Sep 7), [cited January 4, 2015]; 19(52): 47–54. http://search.ebscohost.com/login.aspx?direct=true&db=rzh&AN=106533450&site=ehost-live

[16] Melnyk B, Fineout-Overholt E. *Evidence-based practice in nursing & healthcare: a guide to best practice* [monograph on the Internet]. Philadelphia, Pennsylvania: Lippincott Williams & Wilkins; 2005. http://file.zums.ac.ir/ebook/208-Evidence-Based%20Practice%20in%20Nursing%20&%20Healthcare%20-%20A%20Guide%20to%20Best%20Practice,%20Second%20Edition-Be.pdf

[17] Guideline for management of wounds in patients with lower-extremity venous disease: complete summary [monograph on the Internet]. *U.S. Department of Health and Human Services*. U.S. DepartmentofHealthandHumanServices, 2005. https://www.guideline.gov/summaries/summary/38249/guideline-for-management-of-wounds-in-patients-with-lowerextremity-venous-disease

[18] Forssgren A, Fransson I, Nelzén O. Leg Ulcer Point Prevalence can be Decreased by Broad-scale Intervention: a Follow-up Cross-sectional Study of a Defined Geographical Population*. (Cover story). *Acta Dermato-Venereologica* [serial on the Internet]. (2008, May), [cited January 4, 2015]; 88(3): 252–256. http://search.ebscohost.com/login.aspx?direct=true&db=mnh&AN=18480924&site=ehost-live

[19] Assessment and management of venous leg ulcers: complete summary [monograph on the Internet]. *US National Guideline Clearinghouse* U.S. DepartmentofHealthandHumanServices; 2008. http://www.gacguidelines.ca/site/GAC_Guidelines/assets/pdf/LEGU05-6_Venous_Leg_Ulcer_Summary.pdf

[20] Guideline for management of wounds in patients with lower-extremity arterial disease: complete summary [monograph on the Internet]. *US National Guideline Clearinghouse* U.S. DepartmentofHealthandHumanServices; 2008. https://www.guideline.gov/summaries/summary/38249/guideline-for-management-of-wounds-in-patients-with-lowerextremity-venous-disease

[21] Yarwood-Ross L, Haigh C. Managing a venous leg ulcer in the 21st century, by improving self-care. *British Journal Of Community Nursing* [serial online].

http://dx.doi.org/10.5772/65719

October 2012;17(10):460–465. http://search.ebscohost.com/login.aspx?direct=true&db=rzh&AN=108112049&site=ehost-live

[22] Van Hecke A, Grypdonck M, Defloor T. The clinical nursing competences and their complexity in Belgian general hospitals. *Journal of Advanced Nursing* [serial on the Internet]. 2006;56(6):669–678. [cited January 13, 2011]. http://search.ebscohost.com/login.aspx?direct=true&db=rzh&AN=106290657&site=ehost-live

[23] Domeij D, Flodén M. POPULATION AGING AND INTERNATIONAL CAPITAL FLOWS. *International Economic Review* [serial on the Internet]. (2006, Aug), [cited January 4, 2015]; 47(3): 1013–1032. http://search.ebscohost.com/login.aspx?direct=true&db=bth&AN=21678955&site=ehost-live

[24] Heinen M, Evers A, Van Uden C, CJM, PCM, Van Achterberg T. Sedentary patients with venous or mixed leg ulcers: determinants of physical activity. *Journal of Advanced Nursing* [serial on the Internet]. (2007, Oct), [cited January 4, 2015]; 60(1): 50–57. http://search.ebscohost.com/login.aspx?direct=true&db=rzh&AN=106190961&site=ehost-live

Chapter 6

Aspects Related to Venous Ulcer Healing and its Influence on Quality of Life

Gilson V. Torres, Aline M. Pergola-Marconato, Thalyta C. Mansano-Schlosser, Rhayssa O. Araújo, Dalva C. Silva, Abigail Gómez-Morales, Sandra M.S.G.S.O. Torres, Felismina R.P. Mendes and Eulália M.C. Maia

Additional information is available at the end of the chapter

http://dx.doi.org/10.5772/64913

Abstract

Nowadays, the varicose ulcers (VUs) are one of the most worrying leg ulcers and are an important global health problem, with high costs related to the treatment and its complications. Moreover, the quality of life (QOL) of the patient could be affected by pain, sleep disorders, functional impairment, depression, and isolation. The VU patient care is complex, and it is necessary to know the aspects that contribute to the healing process for developing effective strategies. The members of the multidisciplinary health team should identify sociodemographic, clinical, and care aspects that interfere in tissue repair and therefore impacting the QOL. Self-efficacy, adherence to treatment, and self-esteem are other important aspects also related to healing and QOL, with implications for health care and the multidisciplinary team. To sum up, the use of multidisciplinary protocols allows the systematization of care for people with VUs in order to standardize therapeutic interventions with the aim to decrease the healing process time and, as a consequence, to improve the QOL.

Keywords: wound healing, varicose ulcer, quality of life, self-efficacy, self-concept

INTECH
open science | open minds

1. Introduction

This chapter discusses the aspects related to the healing of venous ulcers (VUs) and its influence on quality of life (QOL), using studies developed in recent years in the Brazilian research group called Nursing Procedures's Incubator Research Group (GPIPE – CNPq) as the main assumptions and corroborating with other national and international references. The understanding of the physiology of a healing chronic wound, as well as the pathophysiology of chronic venous insufficiency (CVI) is fundamental. This is the beginning for the ulceration, allowing members of the multidisciplinary health team to identify sociodemographic, clinical, and care aspects that interfere, directly or indirectly, in tissue repair and therefore impacting the QOL. Other important aspects such as self-efficacy, adherence to treatment, and self-esteem are also related to healing and QOL with implications for health care and the multidisciplinary team.

2. Contextualization of venous ulcer and quality of life

VU is the main lesion of the lower limbs, with an approximate prevalence between 80 and 90%. It is caused by CVI, having an irregular shape, with defined edges, usually located in the perimalleolar region. It is usually limited to the subcutaneous tissue; however, the secondary infection can produce profound destruction of soft tissues [1].

As a chronic wound, it needs prolonged and expensive treatment for the health system and the individual. The healing process has steps that differ from normal wounds and can remain open for a long period. Some of the factors associated with changes in healing are aging, overweight/obesity, nonadherence to compression therapy, extensive, and infection injury area.

People with VU commonly live with chronic pain that can affect the autonomy in carrying out daily activities, decreasing self-esteem, causing social isolation, and depression and thus, interfering in all dimensions of life. It also has a considerable socioeconomic impact due to treatment costs and loss of working days, with the possibility of early retirement.

The World Health Organization (WHO) defines QOL as "the individual's perception of his position in life in the context of culture and value systems in which they live, and about their goals, expectations, standards, and concerns" [2].

There are several generic or specific instruments, which may be used in the evaluation of the person's QOL with VU, such as EuroQol 5 dimensions (EQ-5D), Short Form Health Survey-12 (SF-12); Short Form Health Survey (SF-36), Short Form 6 dimensions (SF-6D), ChronIc Venous Insufficiency Quality of Life Questionnaire (CIVIQ), Cardiff Wound Impact Schedule (CWIS), and Charing Cross Venous Ulcer Questionnaire (CCVUQ).

Thus, its evaluation is important for the understanding of its influence on the healing process and develops effective and secure strategies by health professionals for a comprehensive approach to the patient. The care planning requires the involvement and training of the multidisciplinary team to identify the needs of this population and adequate guidance.

http://dx.doi.org/10.5772/64913

3. Healing physiology and pathophysiology of chronic venous insufficiency and arising of venous ulcers

Healing can be understood as a range of metabolic reactions by the loss of skin integrity, which aim to restore the damaged tissue. The stages of this process are inflammatory or exudative, proliferative, and maturation, resulting in scar formation. The duration of these stages is variable and influenced by factors such as ischemia or poor nutrition and immunesuppression [3].

The chronic wound comes from any cause that delays and prolongs the healing and infection, and local irritation may be associated with this delay. Some theories attempt to explain the extended time, either by excessive degradation of the cell matrix, reduction of proinflammatory mediators or immature fibroblasts. Thus, usually, the re-epithelialization and remodeling of damaged tissue are delayed stages [3].

The CVI is a progressive and debilitating condition that can result in a chronic wound. Vascular and rather a complex origin, it involves etiological multiplicity changing the morfofunctional veins and their valves, compromising the blood flow of the lower limbs [4]. In general, the CVI is a wide range of clinical manifestations of chronic venous disease (CVD) [5].

The development of venous pathology is related to increased venous pressure and impaired blood return of the legs through mechanisms, such as the inefficiency of the calf muscle, venous hypertension, the incompetence of the perforating veins that connect the superficial and deep venous system and failure of the valves, causing blood reflux. Among the factors that determine damage on the veins, there are inflammation, trauma, thromboembolism, surgery, and comorbidities such as obesity, high blood pressure (hypertension), and diabetes [4, 5].

These changes bring several clinical manifestations, from heaviness to ulceration with severe pain. The most common signs and symptoms are dry and irritated skin, itching, swelling, and heaviness in the legs, spatially at the end of the day and typical pain that improves when raising members and it worsens when they are midair and may interfere with ambulation [4]. There are also telangiectasias, varicosities, hyperpigmentation, eczema, lipodermatosclerosis, active or healed ulcers observed [5].

Prolonged venous hypertension associated with valvular incompetence and calf muscle dysfunction promotes microcirculation changes of the lower limbs, resulting in skin changes. The dysfunction of the deep venous system valves is associated with disease progression and VU formation [5].

The red blood cells in the extravascular space, as a result of venous stasis, have a decomposition with consequent release of hemosiderin that causes hyperpigmentation. Furthermore, there may be fibrous tissue deposition in the subcutaneous tissue, resulting in the lipodermatosclerosis. These tissue changes associated with constant venous pressure and blood stasis predisposes to ulceration.

Many additional tests such as ultrasound, Doppler, and angiography, are employed to assist in the diagnosis of CVI and evaluate the venous return. However, there is no diagnostic test that can predict accurately the appearance of VU, which is usually associated with triggering factors such as cellulitis, trauma, dermatitis or skin irritation, insect bites, burns, sudden onset of edemas [4].

VU not showing signs of healing for a time greater than 4–6 weeks may be considered chronic, predisposing to infection, bad odor and pain. Among the reasons for the chronicity of the injury, there is the high concentration of neutrophils that secrete proteases and inhibit the growth factors. Moreover, the presence of fibrin, leukocytes, and microangiopathy contribute to chronic inflammation resulting in changes in the microcirculation, delaying the injury closing. Therefore, infection and antibiotic therapy, topical or systemic, long and low adherence to compression therapy are related to a worse prognosis [4].

VU treatment objectives are the reduction of pain, exudate, odor, and necrotic tissue to prevent the onset of infection. The main interventions are: raising the legs, physical exercise, compression therapy, and the use of dressing coverage [4].

Compressive therapies represent the gold standard treatment for CVI and VU promoting the reduction of venous stasis limiting the distention of the veins and aid in the function of the calf pump. They are contraindicated only in the presence of arterial insufficiency, cellulitis, and decompensate heart failure. Raising the legs is a simple intervention that assists in reducing edema, promoting venous return [4].

The selection of dressing coverage should consider the injury characteristics (tissue, exudate, odor, infection), the patient's needs, such as comfort and allergy, the result of the cost-benefit, and ease of application [4].

Therefore, the participation of a multidisciplinary health team planning and executing comprehensive care is critical. In this team, the nurse plays an essential role in the early identification of manifestations of CVI and the rapid and efficient development of actions that interfere with the progression of the disease and the occurrence of relapses, promoting quality of life [4].

In the case of systematic nursing care for people with VU, a study identified in more than half of the participants, the following factors related to the nursing diagnosis of the North American Nursing Diagnosis Association (NANDA) Impaired tissue integrity: impaired circulation, knowledge deficit, chemical irritants, excess fluids, and nutritional factors [6].

4. Sociodemographic, clinical, and care influence in the healing of venous ulcer and quality of life

As a thought, VU healing receives multifactorial influence beyond the biological aspects. Sociodemographic, clinical, and care characteristics are directly related to this process, also modifying the QOL (**Figure 1**).

http://dx.doi.org/10.5772/64913

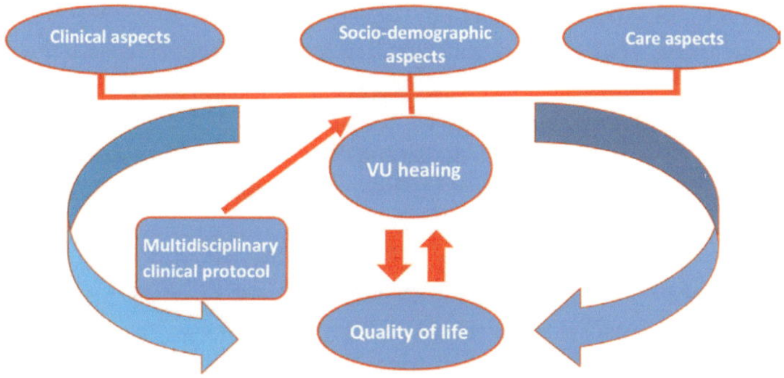

Figure 1. Proposition model of the relationship between the variables interfering with venous ulcer healing and quality of life.

The demographic characteristics of people with VU are similar worldwide. Females, elderly, often with low education, and income are predominant [7–11].

Women are more affected because they are more prone to developing CVI, either for their hormonal activity, the number of pregnancies or even genetic factors. The increase with aging is justified by the incompetence of venous valves, dysfunction of the calf pump due to decreased muscle strength, together with the fragility of the skin, common characteristics in this population.

The low level of education hinders to understand the clinical situation and in promoting health through self-care due to lack of knowledge regarding ulceration, resulting in the absence of lifestyle changes [12, 13].

Income constitutes an important factor because of the high costs of dressing coverage, use of compression therapy, and other care favoring the financial imbalance, often aggravated by leaving the labor activity.

Concerning to clinical and health, the presence of other chronic diseases with CVI, as SAH and DM, as well as health habits, including sleep patterns, alcohol consumption, and smoking are related to the VU healing process.

Diseases such as SAH and DM directly influence blood circulation and healing capacity. Studies show the prevalence and association of these diseases in people with VU [14, 15], which makes them difficult aspects of healing. The hypertension is often associated with atherosclerosis and Diabetes can lead to complications in the skin as a result of neuropathy, also, to often be associated with peripheral arterial disease, making the stabilization of the injury.

Habits such as drinking alcohol and smoking influence the metabolism of the skin, impairing the VU healing process. Nicotine has vasoactive effects, decreasing blood flow, and consequently the amount of oxygen in the tissues [16]. Alcohol drinking is often associated with bad health habits and self-care, damaging the wound closure.

In individuals with VU, one of the clusters symptoms found is the sleep disorder and usually is related to chronic pain, and sleep good quality is essential to strengthen the mental and physical health [17].

Pain is common in this population, with a prevalence of 80–96% of cases. Moreover, it causes physical, emotional and social limitations and tends to be intensified at the time of dressing change or compression therapy [18–20].

In northeastern Brazil, the presence of pain affects QOL and can negatively influence wound healing, being present in 86% of patients [11]. Pain stimulates the release of inflammatory mediators that interfere with repair tissue [21] and, when severe, it can be related to local infection, increasing healing time.

The consequent prolonged injury time also influences the healing and consequently the quality of life. When investigating the association between the VU time, there was worst mean on those people over 1 year of injury, and the emotional state and aesthetics were significantly affected [15]. In another study, the risk factors and pathological personal antecedents were more present in people with treatment time greater than 1 year [22].

As already known, the characteristics of the lesion are directly related to healing. Great and depth injuries with necrosis, lot of fibrin, little granulation tissue, purulent exudate and foul odor naturally lead to a longer time to complete closure.

Care aspects are also directly related to the healing process. Appropriate care has the participation of a multidisciplinary team, preferably with the adoption of protocols, technical skills, and specific knowledge of patient's assessment and injury [10].

The choice and access to the coverage consistent with the tissues shown in the injury as well as the use of compression therapy by the level of vascular insufficiency are aspects of the service that stand out for facilitation of wound healing.

Various therapies may be used together with compression therapy. An almost experimental study with lymphotherapy implementation and compression therapy showed that the intervention group reduced pain and edema, and significantly improve VU healing, confirming the benefits of this treatment [23].

In Brazil, it is very common to use medicinal plants. In general, this care happens before seeking health services or in a complementary way to professional practices. Nursing needs to identify the influence of this popular knowledge in the care of people with venous ulcer [24].

Furthermore, the location for the dressing also can influence this process. In countries with advanced health practices, the dressings are performed in specialized clinics, while in others, they are done at home, often by the individuals with VU or their families/caregivers. This kind of behavior does not allow adequate assistance and contamination-free that can lead to infections in the lesion.

Often, the resolutive treatment of people with VU is done by professionals with expertise in the area or with extensive experience. To direct, organize, and unify the assistance, the use of

http://dx.doi.org/10.5772/64913

protocols is adopted in different settings in the world to reduce the working time and also healing time [25].

It is also important that health professionals record the clinical findings to ensure legal support for the assistance provided, and give continuity of care between professionals and health care levels.

5. Interrelationship among quality of life, self-efficacy, adherence to treatment, self-esteem, and healing of venous ulcer

All factors mentioned above are related to wound healing and therefore to QOL, which is also an influencing agent (**Figure 1**).

This construct is a very common research object in many areas, especially health. Its study related to chronic diseases enables to identify specifics for assessing and proposing new interventions and treatments [9]. Its evaluation in health care is part of the search for a comprehensive view of the individual, who can consider all aspects that may influence the VU healing and the person's QOL.

The QOL of people with VU has already been investigated worldwide because being a chronic wound characteristic, individuals live long with it, and it influences on all aspects of life.

Physical problems are the most issues influencing in this construct, because the injury imposes limitations for various day-to-day activities, and the individual becomes dependent on others. Bathing, dressing, walking, using public transport, performing household activities or activities requiring a little more physical strength become almost impossible for those who live with a VU [10, 26].

Due to the physical limitations arising, these people often become unable to work and help the family income. Depending on the country, in some cases, there is early retirement or benefits by social security.

Regarding the social environment and mental health, the characteristic symptoms of the ulcer as pain, possible fetid odor, lots of exudates, the appearance of dressings, and bandages change the perception of themselves, leading to psychological and social problems. Family relationships between friends and work are affected significantly. Frequenting public places become a dilemma for those people who are concerned about the discomfort they may cause to others [27]. Sexual relationships are also affected, a fact little researched in the scientific area [10, 28].

Thus, support for people with VU, in the various spheres of life is essential and therefore social networks bring benefits to treatment. A qualitative study in southern Brazil, built the following categories: the family is concerned with; I had a lot of help from friends and neighbors, and I do by myself, pointing to the need of the multidisciplinary team, through nursing, knowing this social network and working together with it to strengthen the partnership in care [29].

These findings corroborate another qualitative study that showed the influence of injury in the family and occupational relationships, through three categories: venous ulcer and its impact at work; changes in routine and restrictions on living with venous ulcers; and living with venous ulcers and the need for professional and family care [30].

Another study also developed in southern Brazil composed other categories showing treatment strategies: self-treatment, seek the health service, and religious for pain relief. Study participants reported using simple strategies but limited to pain relief, indicating a gap in care [30].

Therefore, there is an emotional burden that affects aspects related to mental health, emerging feelings of helplessness, coping difficulties, lack of hope with the healing also affecting the set of difficulties in activities of daily living and social isolation [31].

It is noticed that there is an interaction of factors mutually cause and effect impairments in QOL. Physical problems are reflected in the social and mental aspects and vice versa, creating a vicious cycle.

Other constructs with QOL and healing are also investigated, including self-efficacy, adherence to treatment and self-esteem. **Figure 2** demonstrates this interrelationship.

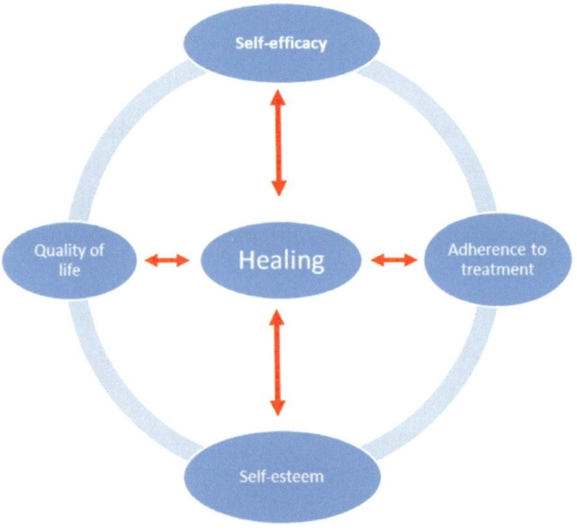

Figure 2. Proposition model of the relationship between the constructs affecting the quality of life and the healing of venous ulcers.

The belief of self-efficacy originated in the Cognitive Social Theory, is the evaluation of what the individual do by himself, based on human motivation, on his ability to perform some activity despite the problems. Thus, self-efficacy is predictive of behavior, which may affect the adaptation and changes in the problems [32, 33].

People acquire beliefs about their abilities from the vicarious experience, social persuasion, somatic and emotional states, and domain experience [33]. Vicarious experience arises from the observation of other people performing tasks [34]. Social persuasion is accomplished through verbal judgments that others do. Somatic and emotional states are anxiety and stress levels influencing the self-confidence level. Finally, the domain experience is obtained from the interpretation of previous actions of the individual [32].

With this understanding, it becomes easy to see how self-efficacy can influence and at the same time be influenced by QOL in people with VU. The existence of injury requires self-care actions such as raising lower limbs, the use of compression therapy and regular physical exercise. These activities will be more effect in people with high self-efficacy, promoting healing, because they interpret the difficult tasks as challenges to be faced, and not as threats to be avoided [33, 34].

The relationship between self-efficacy and chronic diseases is considerably explored, but not specifically at people with VU. However, there is a relationship of self-efficacy with compression therapy and significant association between low self-efficacy and increased risk of recurrence of ulcers [12, 35].

In this sense, self-efficacy is highlighted to improve self-care, QOL, and promoting tissue repair. Professionals can intervene through stimuli to changes in lifestyle, monitoring emotional responses and empowerment for the disease, reducing hopelessness [12, 34, 36].

Therefore, it is necessary to adapt the patients with VU to their new condition of life that affects the mental, physical and social well-being, and generates the search for new skills including values review, knowledge about the disease, adaptation to treatment and facing the society.

With the strong psychosocial impact in this population, health professionals must hold a special care that may reflect an improved QOL, patient's adherence, and self-esteem, providing a high self-efficacy [37, 38].

Therefore, the importance of self-efficacy interference in treatment adherence is highlighted. In a study, it was identified that the level of psychosocial adaptation of these people is low due to the difficulty in treatment adherence, contributing to the chronic nature of these injuries, further compromising QOL [10].

Thus, determined people who are actively involved in the treatment and persist in their goals have high self-efficacy and adapt more easily to their limitations, with a greater chance of success in the faster treatment reestablishment of the physical and psychosocial balance. On the other hand, people with low self-efficacy tend to drop out more easily when not succeed in a particular task, while people with high self-efficacy are more persistent to achieve their goals. Low self-efficacy causes the individual quitting daily activities, social and leisure activities [39].

Therefore, prevention and treatment of VU can be achieved through actions for self-care and self-management programs enable the individuals to manage their health condition regardless of health professionals [40, 41].

Moreover, before that, the therapy adherence is important for people with VU, significantly reducing the healing time, decreasing recurrence rates, and positively influencing QOL [42]. However, it is still a significant problem among people with VU, since the presence of the lesion requires a long, costly treatment, and changes in lifestyle.

Despite the treatment adherence is a problem that deserves the attention of researchers, there are few studies of this nature with the population with VU. In the national context, most studies are done with patients with other chronic diseases.

In a literature review conducted between 2007 and 2012, 69.2% of the studies found a significant relationship between treatment adherence and QOL, but the causality of the phenomenon could not be set. Even on those with no statistical significance, this relationship was positive [43].

Studying the behavior of the patients to treatment is important to understand better the chronic sick person, revealing his greatest difficulties, increasing knowledge about these diseases. Thus, analyzing the phenomenon of adherence is critical to improving health policies and practices aimed at improving the treatment given to the person with VU.

In Brazil, the individual lives with the wound for years. First, because the sociodemographic conditions have disadvantages compared to other countries, and also by the difficult adherence to compression therapy, which also occurs by social issues, as stated earlier. Moreover, the very hot climate of the region does not favor treatment adherence. As there seems to be an effective work of awareness and promotion of compression therapy, treatments are long lasting, expensive and affecting QOL.

Also, high self-esteem acts as a protective factor alleviating the complications related to chronic venous diseases. Thus, damage to self-esteem may adversely affect recovery [44]. In this perspective, evaluating the quality of life and self-esteem is something that has become important in recent decades, specifically, the QOL of patients with venous ulcers, since it is an important indicator of the evolution of response of wound healing [45].

Self-esteem is the personal assessment of the abilities expressed by approving or disapproving attitudes toward himself. This assessment can be carried out globally through the instrument called Rosenberg Self-Esteem Scale [46]. In a recent dissertation, there was a negative and significant correlation between SE of people with VU and domains and dimensions of the SF-36 [47].

6. Implications for health care and the multiprofessional team

From the reflections on the aspects of VU healing and its influence on QOL, the role of health professionals to work in this field is highlighted in this topic.

It is pointed out the relevance of the multidisciplinary health team performance in the multidimensional approach to this population to promote better health outcomes to this population through interventions such as topical therapy, systemic treatment of circulatory conditions, minimizing the impact of injury on self-image, self-esteem, pain management, among others, considering venous ulcer as a chronic injury, recurrent and having a biopsychosocial impact [38, 48, 49].

In this sense, knowing the aspects that impact the QOL of people with VU allows health professionals, especially nurses, incorporating them into the planning of assistance through

http://dx.doi.org/10.5772/64913

interventions that help wound healing. It appears that knowing the situation of individuals, physical and clinical aspects and repercussions on the psychosocial dimensions, nurses can plan actions that meet the care needs to promote better health [38, 49]. Interventions according to clinical presentation and monitoring through systematic evaluation methods are needed [49].

Dressings made by the patients require monitoring and training, to consider aspects of specificity, such as the location of the ulcer, preparation, and receptivity to making the bandage at his home [50, 51]. Thus, the decentralization of care runs through the availability of health staff, especially nurses to conduct training by the treatment cost-benefit and characteristics of the person affected, and each wound [51].

However, there is a weak knowledge and management of nonspecialist nurses on appropriate therapies for the use of topical therapy in the treatment of venous ulcers. The organization and planning of care for nurses are based on the assessment of the ulcer characteristics, as well as the comprehensive approach to people with venous ulcer treatment. By using protocols for topical treatment of VU, it is expected to standardize care, reducing costs and optimizing the nurse's time. Thus, the development of protocols can assist nurses in decision-making on topical therapy [52].

The multidisciplinary protocols allow the systematization of care for people with VU to standardize therapeutic interventions and ensure the continuity of monitoring at various levels of health care. Thus, the healing time and the improvement of QOL decrease [10].

Thus, before the studies in Brazil and discussion with other references throughout this chapter, it is pointed out the need to adopt effective measures that seek to ensure the improvement of QOL of people with VU through a care based on evidence and favoring the integrity of the individual in care.

Author details

Gilson V. Torres[1*], Aline M. Pergola-Marconato[1], Thalyta C. Mansano-Schlosser[1], Rhayssa O. Araújo[1], Dalva C. Silva[1], Abigail Gómez-Morales[1], Sandra M.S.G.S.O. Torres[2], Felismina R.P. Mendes[3] and Eulália M.C. Maia[4]

*Address all correspondence to: gilsonvtorres@hotmail.com

1 Nursing Department at Federal University of Rio Grande do Norte (UFRN), Natal, Brazil

2 Municipal Secretary of Health in Natal, Rio Grande do Norte, Natal, Brazil

3 Nursing School in São João de Deus, Évora University, Évora, Portugal

4 Psychology Department at Federal University of Rio Grande do Norte (UFRN), Natal, Brazil

References

[1] Lal BK. Venous ulcers of the lower extremity: definition, epidemiology, and economic and social burdens. Semin Vasc Surg. 2015;28(1):3–5. DOI: 10.1053/j.semvascsurg. 2015.05.002.

[2] Whoqol Group. The world health organization quality of life assessment (WOQOL): position paper from the world health organization. Soc Sci Med. 1995;11(1):1403–1409.

[3] Dealey C. Fisiologia da cicatrização de feridas. In: Dealey C. Cuidando de feridas: um guia para enfermeiras. São Paulo: Atheneu, 2008. p. 1–12.

[4] Kelechi TJ, Johnson JJ, Yates S. Chronic venous disease and venous leg ulcers: an evidence-based update. J Vasc Nurs. 2015;33(2):36–46. DOI: 10.1016/j.jvn.2015.01.003.

[5] Eberhardt RT, Raffetto JD. Chronic venous insufficiency. Circulation. 2014;130:333–346. DOI: 10.1161/01.CIR.00001641199.72440.08.

[6] Malaquias SG, Bachion MM, Martins MAM, Nunes CAB, Torres GVT et al. Impaired tissue integrity, related factors and defining characteristics in persons with vascular ulcers. Texto & contexto enferm. 2014;23(2):434–442. DOI: 10.1590/0104-07072014001090013.

[7] Evangelista DG, Magalhães ERM, Moretão DIC, Stival MM, Lima LR. Impact of chronic wounds in the quality of life for users of family health strategy. Rev enferm Cent-Oeste Min. 2012;2(2):254–263.

[8] Luz BSR, Atzigen DANCV, Filho MM, Araújo CS, Mendonça ARA, Medeiros ML. Evaluating the effectiveness of the customized Unna boot when treating patients with venous ulcers. An Bras Dermatol. 2013;88(1):41–49. DOI: 10.1590/ S0365-05962013000100004.

[9] Saraiva DMRF, Bandarra AJF, Agostinho ES, Pereira NMM, Lopes TS. Quality of life of service users with chronic venous ulcers. Referência. 2013;3(10):109–118. DOI: 10.12707/ RIII1241.

[10] Costa IKF, Salvetti MG, Souza AJG, Dias TYAF, Dantas DV, Torres GV. Assistance protocol to people with venous ulcers: a methodological study. Online Braz J Nurs. 2015;14(1):05–15. DOI: 10.5935/1676-4285.20154692.

[11] Salvetti MDG, Costa IKF, Dantas DV, Freitas CCSD, Vasconcelos QLDDA, Torres GVT. Prevalence of pain and associated factors in venous ulcer patients. Rev Dor. 2014;15(1): 17–20. DOI: 10.5935/1806-0013.20140005.

[12] Finlayson K, Edwards H, Courtney M. The impact of psychosocial factors on adherence to compression therapy to prevent recurrence of venous leg ulcers. J Clin Nurs. 2010;19(9-10):1289–1297. DOI: 10.1111/j.1365-2702.2009.03151.x.

[13] Heinen MM, Evers AW, Van Uden CJ, Van der Vleuten CJ, van de Kerkhof PC, Van Achterberg T. Sedentary patients with venous or mixed leg ulcers:

determinants of physical activity. J Adv Nurs. 2007;60(1):50–57. DOI: 10.1111/j.1365-2648.2007.04376.x.

[14] Salomé GM, Blanes L, Ferreira LM. The impact of skin grafting on the quality of life and self-esteem of patients with venous leg ulcers. World J Surg. 2014;38(1):233–240. DOI: 10.1007/s00268-013-2228-x.

[15] Araújo RO, Silva DC, Souto RQ, Pergola-Marconato AM, Costa IKF, Torres GV. Impact of varicose ulcers on the quality of life of persons receiving primary care. Aquichan. 2016;16(1):56–66. DOI: 10.5294/aqui.2016.16.1.7.

[16] Sørensen LT, Jørgensen S, Petersen LJ, Hemmingsen U, Bülow J, Loft S et al. Acute effects of nicotine and smoking on blood flow, tissue oxygen, and aerobe metabolism of the skin and subcutis. J Surg Res. 2009;152(2):224–230. DOI: 10.1016/j.jss.2008.02.066.

[17] Edwards H, Finlayson K, Skerman H, Alexander K, Miaskowski C, Aouizerat B et al. Identification of symptom clusters in patients with chronic venous leg ulcers. J Pain Symptom Manage. 2014;47(5):867–875. DOI: 10.1016/j.jpainsymman.2013.06.003.

[18] Gonçalves ML, Gouveia SVL, Pimenta CM, Suzuki E, Komegae KM. Pain in chronic leg ulcers. J Wound Ostomy Continence Nurs. 2004;31(5):275–283.

[19] Oliveira PF, Tatagiba BS, Martins MA, Tipple AF, Pereira LV. Assessment of pain during leg ulcers' dressing change. Texto Contexto Enferm. 2012;21(4):862–869. DOI: 10.1590/S0104-07072012000400017.

[20] Hopman WM, Buchanan M, VanDerkerkhof EG, Harrison MB. Pain and health related quality of life in people with chronic leg ulcers. Chronic Dis Inj Can. 2013;33(3):167–174.

[21] Woo KY, Sibbald RG. The improvement of wound-associated pain and healing trajectory with a comprehensive foot and leg ulcer care model. J Wound Continence Nurs. 2009;36(2):184–191. DOI: 10.1097/01.WON.0000347660.87346.ed.

[22] Torres SMSGSO, Monteiro VGN, Salvetti MG, Melo GSM, Torres GV, Maia EMC. Sociodemographic, clinic and health characterization of people with venous ulcers attended at the family health strategy. Rev Pesqui Cuid Fundam. 2014;6(Suppl.):50–59. DOI: 10.9789/2175-5361.2014.v6i5.50-59.

[23] Azoubel R. Effectiveness of decongestive physical therapy in the healing of venous ulcers [thesis]. Natal: Health Sciences Center, Federal University of Rio Grande do Norte; 2014.

[24] Silva DC, Budó MDLD, Schimith MD, Heisler EV, Simon BS, Torres GVT. Use of medicinal plants by people with venous ulcer in outpatient treatment. Rev Pesqui Cuid Fundam (online). 2015;7(3):2895–2997. DOI: 10.9789/2175-5361.2015.v7i3.2985-2997.

[25] Costa IKF, Nóbrega WG, Costa IKF, Torres GV, Lira ALBC, Tourinho FSV et al. People with venous ulcers: a study of the psychosocial aspects of the adaptive model of Roy. Rev Gauch Enferm. 2011;32(3):561–568. DOI: 10.1590/S1983-14472011000300018.

[26] Lopes CR, Figueiredo M, Ávila AM, Soares LMBM, Dionisio VC. Evaluation of limitations of venous ulcers in legs. J Vasc Bras. 2013;12(1):5–9.

[27] Maddox D. Effects of venous leg ulceration on patients' quality of life. Nurs Stand. 2012;26(38):42–49.

[28] Salomé GM. Living process of a chronic wound carrier: recreational and sexual activities, social and family life. 2010;46(7):300–304.

[29] Silva DCD, Budó MDLD, Schimith M.D, Torres GDV, Durgante VL, Rizzatti SDJS et al. Influence of social networks on the therapeutic itineraries of people with venous ulcer. Rev Gauch Enferm. 2014;35(3):90–96. DOI: 10.1590/1983-1447.2014.03.45072.

[30] Silva DC, Budó MLD, Schimith MD, Ecco L, Costa IKF, Torres GV. Experiences constructed in the process of living with a venous ulcer. Cogitare Enferm. 2015;20(1): 13–19.

[31] Green J, Jester R, McKinley R, Pooler A. The impact of chronic venous leg ulcers: a systematic review. J Wound Care. 2014;23(12):601–612. DOI: 10.12968/jowc. 2014.23.12.601.

[32] Pajares F, Olaz F. Teoria social cognitiva e auto-eficácia: uma visão geral. In: Bandura A, Azzi RB, Polydoro S. Teoria social cognitiva: conceitos básicos. Porto Alegre: Artmed; 2008.

[33] Bandura A. Self-efficacy: toward a unifying theory of behavioral change. Psychol Rev. 1977;84(2):191–215.

[34] Araújo RO. Self-efficacy and quality of life of people with venous ulcers [dissertation]. Natal: Nursing Department, Federal University of Rio Grande do Norte; 2014.

[35] Finlayson K, Edwards H, Courtney M. Relationships between preventive activities, psychosocial factors and recurrence of venous leg ulcers: a prospective study. J Adv Nurs. 2011;67(10):2180–2190. DOI: 10.1111/j.1365-2648.2011.05653.x.

[36] Bonsaksen T, Lerdal A, Fagermoen MS. Factors associated with self-efficacy in persons with chronic illness. Scand J Psychol. 2012;53(4):333–339. DOI: 10.1111/j. 1467-9450.2012.00959.x.

[37] Figueiredo ML, Zuffi FB. Atención a pacientes con úlcera venosa: percepción de los enfermeros de Estrategia de Salud Familiar. Enferm Glob. 2012;28:147–158.

[38] Silva FAA, Moreira TMM. Sociodemografic and clinical characteristics of customers with venous leg ulcer. Rev Enferm UERJ. 2011;19(3):468–472.

[39] Salvetti MG, Pimenta CAM, Braga PE, Corrêa CF. Disability related to chronic low back pain: prevalence and associated factors. Rev Esc Enferm USP. 2012;46(esp):16–23. DOI: 10.1590/S0080-62342012000700003.

[40] Costa LM, Higino WJ, Leal FDJ, Couto RC. Clinical and socio-demographic profile of patients with venous disease treated in health centers of Maceió (AL), Brazil. J Vasc Bras. 2012;11(2):108–113. DOI: 10.1590/S1677-54492012000200007.

[41] Brown A, Kendall S, Flanagan M, Cottee M. Encouraging patients to selfcare – the preliminary development and validation of the VeLUSET©, a self-efficacy tool for venous leg ulcer patients, aged 60 years and over. Int Wound J. 2014;11(3):326–334.

[42] Bistreanu R, Teodorescu M. Venous leg ulcer–patient compliance to treatment and impact on quality of life. J Exp Med Surg Res. 2009;XVI(2):97–102.

[43] Liberato SMD, Souza AJGS, Gomes ATLG, Medeiros LPM, Costa IKF, Torres GVT. Relationship between treatment adherence and quality of life: integrative literature review. Rev Eletrônica Enferm. 2014;16(1):191–198. DOI: 10.5216/ree.v16i1.22041.

[44] Hutz CS, Zanon C. Revision of the adaptation, validation, and normatization of the Roserberg self-esteem scale. Aval Psicol. 2011;10(1):41–49.

[45] Salomé GM, Blanes L, Ferreira LM. Evaluation of depressive symptoms in patients with venous ulcers. Rev Bras Cir Plást. 2012;27(1):124–129. DOI: 10.1590/S1983-51752012000100021.

[46] Santos PJ, Maia J. Confirmatory factor analysis and preliminary validation of a Portuguese version of the Rosenberg self-esteem scale. Psychology: Theory, research and practice. 2003;(2):253–268.

[47] Souza AJG. Self-esteem and quality of life of people with venous ulcers treated in the primary care [dissertation]. Natal: Nursing Department, Federal University of Rio Grande do Norte; 2014.

[48] Torres GVT, Costa IKF, Silva RKSM, Oliveira AKA, Souza AJG, Mendes FRP. The characterization of persons with venous ulcer in Brazil and Portugal: comparitive study. Enferm Glob. 2013;12(32):62–74.

[49] Sant'Ana SMSC, Bachion MM, Santos QR, Nunes CAB, Malaquias SG, Oliveira BGRB. Venous ulcers: clinical characterization and treatment in users treated in outpatient facilities. Rev Bras Enferm. 2012;65(4):637–644. DOI: 10.1590/S0034-71672012000400013.

[50] Brito CKD, Nottingham IC, Victor JF, Feitoza SMS, Silva MG, Amaral HEG. Venous ulcer: clinical assessment, guidelines and dressing care. Rev RENE. 2013;14(3):470–480.

[51] Oliveira SB, Soares DA, Pires PS. Prevalence of venous ulcers and associated factors among adults of a health center in Vitória da Conquista – BA. Rev Pesqui Cuid Fundam. 2015;7(3):2659–2669. DOI: 10.9789/2175-5361.2015.v7i3.2659-2669.

[52] Sellmer D, Carvalho CMG, Carvalho DR, Malucelli A. Expert system to support the decision in topical therapy for venous ulcers. Rev Gaucha Enferm. 2013;34(2):154–162. DOI: 10.1590/S1983-14472013000200020.

Chapter 7

Placental Cells and Tissues: The Transformative Rise in Advanced Wound Care

Jeremy J. Lim and Thomas J. Koob

Additional information is available at the end of the chapter

http://dx.doi.org/10.5772/65321

Abstract

The fetal environment has a remarkable capacity for facilitating and guiding tissue development. Placental tissues including the placental disc, umbilical cord, amniotic fluid and amniotic sac are highly specialized tissues responsible for transporting nutrients and coordinating developmental cues during pregnancy and fetal development. Placental tissues are nutrient-rich, structurally complex and immunologically privileged, making them promising allograft therapies for advanced wound care. Amniotic membrane allografts in particular have been shown to be effective therapies for treatment of chronic wounds, including diabetic and venous ulcers, by modulating inflammation, reducing scar tissue formation and enhancing healing. Amniotic membrane has also demonstrated the ability to promote cell proliferation, cell migration and modulate cytokine secretion by a variety of cell types involved in wound healing, including human dermal fibroblasts, microvascular endothelial cells and stem cells. In addition, amniotic membrane allografts have been shown to stimulate stem cell activity, promote angiogenesis and modulate inflammation *in vitro* and *in vivo*. Placental tissues are complex tissues composed of extracellular matrix (ECM), cells and a broad array of cytokines that may collectively enhance wound healing by modulating wound environments and stimulating endogenous cells to progress through the normal healing stages of inflammation, proliferation and remodeling.

Keywords: placenta, umbilical cord, amniotic fluid, amniotic membrane, dHACM

1. Introduction

The fetal environment has a remarkable capacity for facilitating and guiding tissue development. Starting from a single fertilized egg, fetal cells proliferate, migrate, differentiate and respond to local and external environmental cues to develop into a fully healthy human body, including musculoskeletal, neural and cardiovascular systems. The fetal environment is critical in embryogenesis and fetal development, as the maternal environment provides specific cues for development and fetal cells respond to those maternal cues. This remarkable sequence of signals guides cell cleavage and differentiation throughout gestation in a spatially and temporally coordinated fashion.

In particular, the placenta is a highly specialized organ that develops as a conduit between maternal and fetal tissues with the primary function of transporting nutrients and developmental signals between the mother and the fetus. The placenta is composed of four distinct tissues, as depicted in **Figure 1**, including:

- placental disc,
- umbilical cord,
- amniotic fluid and
- amniotic sac or membrane.

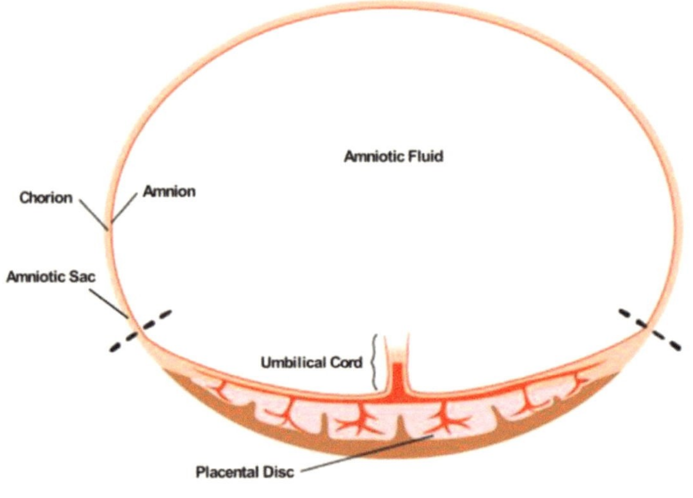

Figure 1. Placental tissues include the placental disc, umbilical cord, amniotic fluid and amniotic sac. The amniotic sac is composed of the amnion and chorion layers.

The placental disc connects the blood supply of the developing fetus with the mother to regulate nutrition, waste removal, hormonal balance and the immune system, while also acting as an immunologically privileged barrier to prevent direct contact between the maternal and fetal blood [1]. Placental tissues including the umbilical cord, amniotic fluid and amniotic sac play significant roles in regulating tissue development by maintaining the fetal environment. The developing fetus receives nutrients from the placenta through the umbilical cord vessels and the fetus is continually bathed in amniotic fluid, which cushions and protects the fetus. The amniotic fluid is physically contained and biologically regulated by the amniotic sac, which secretes regulatory proteins and signals into the amniotic fluid and to the fetus. Together these placental tissues, including the placental disc, umbilical cord, amniotic fluid and amniotic sac, provide nutrition, protect the fetus and act as an immunologically privileged barrier to regulate fetal development.

Due to their role in tissue development, placental tissues are nutrient-rich and structurally complex tissues, which have been investigated as advanced wound care therapies. Additionally, fetal tissues are immunologically privileged [2] and the placenta is normally discarded after birth, making placental tissues an available source of donor tissue with low risk of immunological rejection. Placental tissues, including amniotic membrane, umbilical cord, amniotic fluid and placental disc, have rapidly escalated in use as allografts to enhance healing of wounds. These placental allografts are naturally derived tissues composed of cells, extracellular matrix (ECM) and a complex array of regulatory cytokines with the inherent function of supporting tissue growth and modulating inflammation. Amniotic membrane allografts in particular have been shown to be effective therapies for healing of chronic wounds, including diabetic and venous ulcers [3, 4]. Placental tissues have also demonstrated the ability to promote cell proliferation, cell migration and modulate cytokine secretion by a variety of cell types involved in wound healing, including human dermal fibroblasts, microvascular endothelial cells and stem cells [5–8]. This chapter will provide a review of placental tissues and their role in wound healing.

Published literature was reviewed for *in vitro, in vivo* and clinical studies on the use of placental tissues for wound care and soft tissue healing. Databases such as PubMed, Google Scholar and Google Books were searched for terms relevant to the structure, function and biomedical application of placental tissues, including the amniotic membrane, umbilical cord, amniotic fluid and placental disc and various review articles and citations were used to identify applicable publications. Where appropriate, discussion was primarily limited to recently published, peer-reviewed studies and completed randomized controlled clinical trials to focus on high quality research.

2. Role of placental cells and tissues in fetal development

2.1. Placental development

The placenta is a remarkable organ with very unique characteristics, including being a nutrient-rich and immunologically privileged tissue. The structure and function of the placenta during pregnancy and fetal development gives placental tissues unique characteristics that can be utilized to enhance healing of wounds. The placental disc is composed of both maternally- and fetally-derived tissues to form a specialized maternal/fetal barrier that facilitates transport between maternal and fetal blood without direct contact. The fetal component of the placenta, called the chorion frondosum, develops from the fetal blastocyst, while the maternal component, called the decidua basalis, develops from the maternal uterine tissue. Placental development is initiated after fertilization and implantation.

Upon fertilization, an egg undergoes cleavage, cavitation and differentiation to form a multicellular structure called a blastocyst. A blastocyst is composed of an inner cell mass, which contains embryonic stem cells that become the embryo and an outer cell layer that is called the trophoblast. As a part of the female menstrual cycle, the maternal uterus undergoes a process called decidualization in response to hormonal changes, including cyclic secretion of 17β-estradiol and progesterone [1]. The maternal endometrium subsequently undergoes remodeling, which includes increased glandular epithelial secretion, influx of specialized uterine natural killer cells and vascular remodeling, to prepare itself for blastocyst implantation [9].

After the blastocyst implants into the maternal endometrium, the trophoblast develops to form the outer layer of the placenta. Trophoblast cells rapidly proliferate and differentiate to form an inner layer of cytotrophoblast cells and the cytotrophoblast cells differentiate and fuse to form an outer multinucleated syncytiotrophoblast cell layer that covers the placenta. The syncytiotrophoblast extends into the endometrial epithelium and invades the connective tissue, as the blastocyst sinks beneath the endometrial surface. Lacunar networks form within the syncytiotrophoblast, allowing maternal blood to flow in and out of the networks and extensions of proliferating cytotrophoblasts evaginate into the syncytiotrophoblast forming the chorionic villi of the placenta [1]. As the placenta develops, the trophoblast layers form a placental barrier, where a layer of cells separate the maternal blood in the intervillous space from the fetal blood in the villi.

In response to blastocyst implantation, the maternal endometrium undergoes a decidual reaction in which the decidual stromal cells accumulate glycogen and nutrients and increase secretory function to support the early embryo [1]. Also, decidualizing stromal cells acquire the unique ability to regulate trophoblast invasion, to resist inflammatory and oxidative insults and to dampen local maternal immune responses. Stromal cells increase expression of various factors including prolactin, insulin-like growth factor binding protein 1 (IGFBP-1), tissue factor, interleukin 15 (IL-15) and vascular endothelial growth factor (VEGF) [9].

As the maternal uterine endometrium undergoes decidualization, the spiral arteries in the decidua are remodeled to become less convoluted and larger to increase maternal blood flow to the placenta. Maternal vessels are disrupted to form the intervillous space, where maternal blood comes in direct contact with fetal chorion frondosum, though no fluid is exchanged across the membrane.

2.2. Placental structure and composition

The intervillous space lies in between the fetal chorionic villi and the maternal blood vessels and contains the main functional units of the placenta. In the intervillous space, extensively branched and closely packed villous structures contain fetal blood vessels. The intervillous space is lined with syncytiotrophoblasts and at this border, maternal blood enters via spiral endometrial arteries [1]. To support blood flow and nutrient transport, the relatively high pressure of maternal blood fills the intervillous space of the placenta and bathes the fetal villi in blood. Maternal-fetal exchange of nutrients occurs at the terminal regions of the chorionic

http://dx.doi.org/10.5772/65321

villi. Then as the maternal blood pressure decreases, the deoxygenated blood drains out of the intervillous space into the maternal bloodstream through the endometrial veins.

In the fetal circulation, the umbilical cord connects the fetal blood to the placental circulation. The umbilical cord connects to the chorionic plate of the placental disc and the vessels branch radially over the surface of the placenta to form a network of villous tree structures [1]. The umbilical vessels branch in the placenta to form chorionic vessels, which then branch again to form cotyledon vessels. These vessels in the chorionic villi form an extensive network, which brings fetal blood extremely close to maternal blood with no intermingling. In the intervillous space, maternal and fetal blood come as close as 2–4 μm of each other to facilitate transport across the placental barrier without direct contact or mixing of blood [1]. As a result, signals and nutrients in the maternal and fetal blood become intertwined throughout pregnancy.

Given the unique function of the placenta, it is no surprise that placental tissue components, including ECM, cells and cytokines, are intricately organized. These bioactive tissue matrices can be used for a variety of medical applications, including treatment of wounds, especially when the biological components of the tissues are preserved.

2.2.1. Placental disc

The placental disc is composed of a highly vascularized extracellular matrix. Collagens I, III, IV and VI have been identified in the placental disc, with collagen type I being the predominant structural component [10]. Additionally, the placenta disc contains a vast distribution of noncollagenous glycoproteins and proteoglycans, including fibronectin, fibrillin I, laminin, thrombospondin I, tenascin C, decorin, heparan sulfate proteoglycans and elastin [11]. This distribution of diverse ECM components can influence cellular differentiation, hormone and protein production, proteolytic activity, as well as various repair mechanisms. Of note, collagen IV, laminin and heparan sulfate, which are normally associated with basement membranes in most adult organs, are expressed weakly throughout the villous stroma and this distribution may facilitate remodeling of basement membranes and increase morphogenetic and functional flexibility of various villous cell populations [10].

The various cell types in the placental disc include trophoblasts, connective tissue fibroblasts, vascular cells, as well as a population of placental mesenchymal stem cells (MSCs) [12]. Due to the role of the placenta in nutrient transport, the placenta is also rich in a number of nutrients and cytokines, including water, electrolytes, vitamins, glucose, proteins, amino acids, lipids and triglycerides. However, because the placental disc contains maternally derived tissue, placental disc tissue typically requires complete decellularization to remove immunological components and use for transplantation is limited to the extracellular matrix.

2.2.2. Umbilical cord

In addition to the placental disc, other placental tissues include the umbilical cord, amniotic sac and amniotic fluid, which are derived from fetal tissues and also have unique structures and functions to support pregnancy and development.

The umbilical cord is composed of Wharton's jelly, which surrounds the umbilical vein and umbilical arteries, contained by an epithelium. The umbilical vein carries oxygenated, nutrient-rich blood from the placenta to the fetus and two umbilical arteries return deoxygenated blood and waste products away from the fetus to the placenta. The umbilical cord connects to the fetal blood supply through the abdomen which will become the navel after birth and within the fetus, the umbilical vein carries oxygenated blood to the hepatic portal vein which carries blood to the liver and the inferior vena cava which carries blood to the heart. The fetal internal iliac arteries then connect to the two umbilical arteries to return deoxygenated blood back into the umbilical cord toward the placenta.

Wharton's jelly is a gelatinous substance composed largely of a diffuse ECM that is rich in collagen and hyaluronic acid, as well as low cellularity of fibroblasts. Collagens I, III, V and VI form an insoluble collagen fibril network, along with an interpenetrating glycoprotein network of fibrillin-rich microfibrils [13, 14]. Hyaluronic acid, the predominant glycosaminoglycan in Wharton's jelly, is immobilized within the insoluble network, forming a hydrated gel that maintains the tissue architecture of the cord and protects the umbilical vessels from extension and compression [15, 16]. The umbilical cord also contains lower amounts chondroitin sulfate, dermatan sulfate, keratin sulfate and heparan sulfate proteoglycans [13].

The Wharton's jelly contains a population of stromal fibroblast-like and myofibroblast-like cells, along with a population of MSCs [15]. Though cell density in the umbilical cord is relatively sparse, these cells are encased in a high volume of ECM suggesting that umbilical cord cells are responsible for secreting large amounts of ECM in order to maintain the tissue matrix [16]. Wharton's jelly also acts as a reservoir of growth factors, which are bound to high molecular weight ECM components. The Wharton's jelly contains acidic fibroblast growth factor (aFGF), basic fibroblast growth factor (bFGF), epidermal growth factor (EGF), insulin-like growth factor 1 (IGF-I), IGFBPs, platelet-derived growth factor (PDGF), transforming growth factor α (TGF-α) and TGF-β [15, 16] and these growth factors and cytokines control cell proliferation and differentiation, protein synthesis and remodeling of the ECM.

2.2.3. Amniotic sac

The human amniotic sac is a thin membrane that contains the amniotic fluid and holds the developing fetus. The amniotic sac comprises two distinct but conjoined membranes—the amnion and chorion. The amnion comprises the inner surface nearest the fetus and contacts the amniotic fluid, while the chorion is nearest the uterus. The membranes consist of an organized collagen-rich ECM, various cells and an abundance of regulatory proteins and signaling molecules. The amnion is composed of an epithelium, followed by a basement membrane, compact layer and fibroblast layer. The epithelium, which faces the developing fetus, consists of a single layer of epithelial cells uniformly arranged on the basement membrane. The basement membrane is a thin layer composed of collagens III and IV and noncollagenous glycoproteins laminin, nidogen and fibronectin [17]. The compact layer is a dense layer almost totally devoid of cells and forms the main fibrous structure of the amnion. Interstitial collagens I and III form bundles in the compact layer that maintain the mechanical integrity of the membrane, while collagens V and VI form filamentous connections to the basement membrane [17]. The fibroblast layer consists of fibroblasts embedded in a loose collagen network with islands of noncollageneous glycoproteins [18].

An intermediate, or spongy, layer separates the amnion and chorion membranes. A nonfibrillar meshwork of collagen III and an abundance of proteoglycans and glycoproteins form a loosely connected jelly-like structure that is high in water content [17, 19]. The intermediate layer acts as an interface that allows the amnion and chorion to glide over one another.

The chorion layer is three to four times thicker than the amnion. Chorion is composed of a reticular layer, pseudobasement membrane and trophoblast layer [17]. The reticular layer contacts the intermediate layer and is composed of collagens I, III, IV, V and VI [17, 20]. The pseudobasement membrane anchors the trophoblasts to the reticular layer with collagen IV, fibronectin and laminin [17, 20]. The trophoblast layer faces the maternal tissue and consists of 2–10 layers of trophoblasts [20]. The trophoblast layer of the chorion frondosum is adhered to the maternal decidua on the surface of the placental disc; however, in the amniotic sac, the chorion does not integrate with decidual tissue.

The amnion and chorion contain no blood vessels and have no direct blood supply; thus, required nutrients are supplied to the amniotic membranes directly through diffusion out of the amniotic fluid or from the underlying decidua [19]. Likewise, the membranes also secrete substances both into the amniotic fluid and toward the uterus, influencing both amniotic fluid homeostasis and maternal cellular physiology, respectively [1]. To date, 226 growth factors, cytokines, chemokines and regulatory proteins have been identified in amniotic membrane-derived tissues [21]. These molecules include growth factors, immunomodulatory cytokines and chemokines and tissue inhibitors of metalloproteinases (TIMPs), such as PDGF-AA, PDGF-BB, TGF-α, TGF-β, bFGF, EGF, VEGF, IL-10, IL-4, placental growth factor (PlGF), TIMP-1, TIMP-2 and TIMP-4, which possess important regulatory roles in regulating fetal development and pregnancy [5].

2.2.4. *Amniotic fluid*

Amniotic fluid surrounds and bathes the fetus during development. Amniotic fluid is generated from the maternal plasma, which passes through the amniotic membranes through osmotic and hydrostatic forces. Early in development, amniotic fluid has a similar composition to fetal plasma and is absorbed through the fetal skin, amniotic membrane, placental surface and umbilical cord [22]. After keratinization of the fetal skin, the fluid is primarily absorbed by the fetus through breathing and swallowing of the amniotic fluid. The amniotic fluid is also exchanged through fetal urination and secretion of oral, nasal, tracheal and pulmonary fluids. Amniotic fluid is predominantly composed of water and contains carbohydrates, proteins, lipids, electrolytes, fetal waste products such as urea and meconium and low numbers of a heterogeneous population of fetal-derived cells.

The volume of amniotic fluid increases during pregnancy up to a peak volume of 800 mL by 28 weeks as the fetus grows, in order to cushion and protect the developing fetus. Near term, the volume declines to approximately 400 mL [22]. Despite a continual flow of fluid between the fetus and placenta, the volume and composition of the amniotic fluid are highly controlled by various mechanisms. Hyaluronic acid is the primary extracellular matrix component that is suspended with the amniotic fluid. Hyaluronic acid increases the viscosity of amniotic fluid, supporting lubrication and movement within the amniotic sac. Hyaluronic acid may also play an important role in fetal healing, which is known to lack fibrous scarring, since hyaluronic acid is deposited early in the healing process in adult tissues and is also known to interact with a variety of growth factors and signaling molecules during the wound healing process [23].

The amniotic fluid is rich in a number of key signaling molecules that play critical roles in fetal development. Amniotic fluid contains a variety of growth factors, carbohydrates, proteins, lipids, electrolytes and other nutrients, including high levels of EGF, TGF-α, TGF-β, IGF-I, erythropoietin (EPO), granulocyte colony-stimulating factor (GCSF) and macrophage colony-stimulating factor (MCSF) [22]. As a key regulator of the fetal innate immune system, amniotic fluid also contains a variety of enzymes, antimicrobial peptides and immunomodulatory mediators that protect the fetus from infection [22, 24]. Amniotic fluid contains a low cellularity of heterogeneous fetal-derived cell types, including epithelial cells from the fetal skin and amnion membrane, cells from the digestive, respiratory and urogenital tracts, as well as a small population of multipotent stem cells [25].

2.3. Stem cells derived from placental tissues

Placental tissues, including the amniotic fluid, amniotic membrane and umbilical cord, are a rich source of multipotent stem cells with the ability to differentiate down multiple lineages and possessing potent immunomodulatory properties. Placental stem cells include hematopoietic and mesenchymal stem cells. Because placental stem cells can be derived from a readily available source of tissue that involves minimal ethical concerns, placental stem cells present significant promise as a cell-based therapy to treat disease [25].

The amniotic membrane contains several populations of multipotent cells, which include amniotic epithelial cells (AECs), amnion-derived MSCs and chorion-derived MSCs [26]. AECs express surface markers that are characteristic of embryonic stem cells, such as stage-specific embryonic antigen 3 (SSEA-3), SSEA-4, TRA-1-60 and TRA-1-81, as well as transcription factors that are commonly associated with pluripotent stem cells, including Oct-4 and Nanog [27]. AECs can give rise to cells in all three germ layers. AECs express nonclassical human leukocyte antigen G (HLA-G), but low levels of HLA-A and -B antigens suggesting that they are immunologically inert [19, 26]. The amnion and chorion are also a source of amniotic membrane stem cells that closely resemble MSCs. Amniotic membrane MSCs (AM-MSCs) express surface markers and differentiation potential consistent with bone marrow MSCs and also express low levels of HLA-A and -B [28].

The amniotic fluid also contains a population of multipotent stem cells. Similar to AM-MSCs, amniotic fluid stem cells (AFSCs) are phenotypically similar to bone marrow MSCs and possess similar multilineage potential [25, 29]. AFSCs may be derived from fetal tissue or multipotent cells from the amniotic membrane. AFSCs also retain some characteristics of embryonic stem cells like expression of SSEA-4 and Oct-4 and differentiation potential down all the three germ lineages [25, 29], suggesting that AFSCs are an intermediate cell type between embryonic stem cells and adult mesenchymal stem cells [30].

http://dx.doi.org/10.5772/65321

Umbilical cord blood is known to be a rich source of hematopoietic stem cells (HSCs) and MSCs [31]; however, Wharton's jelly also acts as a niche, which contains umbilical cord stem cells (UCSCs). UCSCs express similar phenotypic surface markers and differentiation potential to bone marrow MSCs [15, 32].

Placental-derived MSCs possess potent immunomodulatory and reparative properties [26, 33]. Therefore, placental-derived MSCs have been investigated clinically and preclinically for regeneration of tissues and treatment of a variety of diseases and disorders, including treatment of dermal wounds [25, 26, 34, 35]; however, to date live cell therapies have demonstrated limited clinical efficacy due to limited viability and engraftment, as well as phenotypic changes involved with expansion and cryopreservation of live cells [36–39].

2.4. Placental function

By supplying nutrients to the fetus without direct mixing of maternal and fetal blood that could lead to immunological rejection, the placenta plays a key role in supporting fetal development. Through the unique structure of the placental tissues, the placenta connects the developing fetus to the maternal blood supply to provide thermoregulation, nutrient exchange, waste elimination, as well as immunological and physical protection.

2.4.1. Nutrient and waste transport

Perfusion of blood through the placental disc allows transfer of critical nutrients and oxygen from the maternal blood to the fetal circulation. The umbilical cord and vessels connect the fetal blood supply to the placenta and facilitate delivery of nutrients to the developing fetus. Transport occurs through passive diffusion of soluble components across the placental membrane, as well as active transport, which requires expenditure of energy. The placenta transports a full array of nutrients from maternal to fetal blood to support fetal development. The placenta controls transport of water, electrolytes, vitamins, glucose, proteins, amino acids, lipids and triglycerides through both active and passive mechanisms [1]. Many nutrients are present in similar concentrations in fetal and maternal blood and can travel across the placental membranes by simple diffusion down a concentration gradient. However, some nutrients are required in higher concentrations in fetal blood than in the maternal plasma to support fetal development. Therefore, these nutrients require active transport across the placental membrane to concentrate these molecules in fetal blood against a concentration gradient.

The placental membrane is highly permeable to respiratory gases, including rapid diffusion of oxygen from the maternal to fetal blood and of carbon dioxide from fetal to maternal blood. In fact, fetal hemoglobin has a higher affinity for oxygen and lower affinity for carbon dioxide than maternal hemoglobin, which supports favorable gas exchange between the fetal and maternal blood [1]. Transport of water across the placental membrane occurs readily by hydrostatic forces and osmotic pressure and electrolyte balance within the fetal plasma is critical to the function of cellular environments. Ions such as sodium and chloride are present in similar levels in fetal and maternal blood and transport occurs largely by passive diffusion. However, some ion levels including potassium, magnesium, calcium and phosphate are generally higher in fetal blood than maternal plasma, indicating that they undergo active transport across the placental membrane via a number of ion pumps and transporters [1].

Glucose is a critical carbohydrate transported across the placenta and is the primary source of energy for the fetus. Glucose is transported across the placental membrane by facilitated diffusion through protein channels and glucose transporters [1]. Amino acids, which are the building blocks that make up proteins, are generally more abundant in fetal plasma than in maternal plasma, indicating that amino acids undergo active transport across the placental membrane [1]. Lipid transport across the placenta includes free fatty acids, triglycerides, phospholipids, glycolipids, sphingolipids, cholesterol, cholesterol esters, fat-soluble vitamins and other compounds. These lipids remain bound to water-soluble lipoproteins in plasma and are transported by active and passive mechanisms.

Along with the transport of nutrients, the placenta also supports removal of waste products from the fetal blood including urea, uric acid, creatinine and carbon dioxide back to the maternal blood [1]. Due to the immature fetal liver, the placenta is also responsible for breaking down various waste products through endogenous enzymes and transport proteins involved in the handling of bile acids, biliary pigments and xenobiotics and for transporting waste products to the maternal blood where they are processed and removed from the maternal circulation by the maternal liver and kidney [40].

2.4.2. Endocrine secretion

Beyond transport between the mother and child, the placenta also acts as an endocrine organ by producing hormones and steroids. The mother's hormone levels change throughout pregnancy and the placenta secretes various hormones essential to support pregnancy and fetal development, including estrogen, progesterone, chorionic gonadotrophin, placental lactogen and placenta growth hormone [1]. These hormones control different aspects of the maternal reproductive organs, uterine contraction, placental development, metabolism, cell differentiation and fetal development. The placenta also produces a large number of growth factors including EGF, IGF and PDGF, as well as various cytokines, chemokines, eicosanoids, vasoactive autacoids and others to support pregnancy and development.

The amniotic membrane also sends signals to the fetus through the amniotic fluid and to the mother through the uterus. In addition to physically encasing the amniotic fluid and developing fetus, the amniotic membrane is a bioactive tissue that plays an integral biological role in fetal development and progression of pregnancy through secretion of growth factors, cytokines, chemokines and related regulatory factors produced by endogenous cells. Therefore, the amniotic membrane and amniotic fluid harbor significant biological activity, including a significant number of developmental cytokines that play important roles in tissue formation.

2.4.3. Fetal immunity

The placenta also plays critical roles in supporting fetal immunity. The placenta and amniotic membrane fight against infection by acting as a selective barrier to inhibit transmission of certain microbes, including bacteria, viruses and xenobiotics. The placenta, amniotic fluid and amniotic membrane also contain a number of enzymes that metabolize drugs and xenobiotics, as well as antimicrobial effectors and immunomodulatory mediators that protect the fetus from infection [22, 41]. Additionally, the placenta permits transport of IgG antibodies from the maternal plasma to support passive immunity in the fetus by providing a copy of maternal humoral immunity [1].

The placental barrier is also critical to preventing immunological rejection of the fetal tissues by the maternal immune system, as the trophoblast layers come in direct contact with maternal decidua and blood, including maternal natural killer (NK) cells and macrophages, but are not rejected. Though the various mechanisms for immune tolerance remain under investigation, the syncytiotrophoblast and cytotrophoblast lack HLA-A and -B tissue antigens, while expressing HLA-C, -E, -F and -G antigens. Absence of classical HLA-A and -B antigens likely prevent recognition by cytotoxic T cells, while the presence of nonclassical HLA-G antigens is necessary to prevent destruction by maternal NK cells. HLA-C is the only classical MHC Class I antigen expressed and HLA-G in particular does not distinguish between individuals but may support antiviral, immunosuppressive and nonimmunological functions [42]. Similarly, as a biological barrier between the mother and child, amniotic membrane tissues naturally contain low levels of HLA-A and -B antigens and β2-microglobulin and are therefore considered immunologically privileged tissues.

The placental trophoblasts also secrete an array of signals that inhibit cytotoxic T cells in the maternal decidua, including Fas ligand, indoleamine-2,3-dioxygenase (IDO), vasoactive intestinal peptide (VIP), phosphocholine, programmed death ligand 1 (PDL1) and progesterone [2, 43]. These signals interact with NK cells, helper T cells and regulatory T cells to suppress immune responses [2, 43]. Therefore, placental tissues have immunologically privileged properties, which make them a promising source of allograft tissue for treatment of wounds.

2.4.4. Protection and cushioning

Amniotic fluid physically cushions the fetus within the mother's abdomen, while allowing fetal movement and promoting musculoskeletal development [22]. The fetus and amniotic fluid are enclosed within the amniotic membrane, which acts as a mechanically robust barrier between the mother and the child. This thin membrane must possess the structural integrity to support the pregnancy through term. Therefore, the amniotic membrane is a metabolically active tissue, which continually remodels and grows to accommodate the increasing volume of the conceptus and amniotic fluid without premature rupture.

3. History of placental tissues for wound healing

Placental tissues including umbilical cord, amniotic sac and amniotic fluid are nutrient-rich tissues that support fetal development and are immunologically privileged to prevent rejection by the maternal immune system. These characteristics make them promising tissues to support wound healing. Though the complex cascade of signals involved in tissue development is not fully understood to date, placental tissues are able to control and regulate the proper balance of many factors to facilitate growth of the embryo. Therefore, the placenta may contain specific regulatory signals that may be critical for tissue growth and these signals may also provide a unique stimulus to promote healing of complex wounds in adults.

At birth, the placenta separates from the wall of the uterus and is expelled from the body. The mother and child no longer require the function of the placenta to facilitate nutrient transport and pregnancy after birth. The umbilical cord is cut from the child and placental tissues are typically discarded as medical waste. Therefore, placental tissues are a plentiful source of donor tissue with significant potential for use as allografts. These tissues are rich in nutrients and the fetal components of the placenta possess significant immunological properties, which make them ideal tissues to promote wound healing.

3.1. Early evidence of efficacy

Placental tissue has been used as allografts since the early twentieth century. In particular, amniotic membrane tissue has been shown to promote healing in a variety of applications including wounds, ophthalmology and surgery [44]. Amniotic membrane allografts have a number of naturally inherent properties that make them beneficial tissues to promote healing. The amniotic membrane tissue provides a natural barrier and ECM scaffold for wound healing and the amniotic membrane also contains an abundance of various growth factors and biological macromolecules important in regulating the physiological healing response [5]. The natural composition of amniotic membrane gives the tissue the biological activity to enhance healing, modulate inflammation and reduce scar formation.

The first reported use of amniotic membrane for skin transplantation was in 1910 [45]. A variety of cases followed including reconstructive OB/GYN surgery, dentistry, neurosurgery and general surgical applications with reports of decreased pain, low rates of infection and improved healing [44]. In the 1940s, promising outcomes were reported for use in healing of the ocular surface [46] and beginning in the 1960s, use of amniotic membrane as wound coverings for treatment of burns and chronic wounds increased [47].

Despite promising results indicating that amniotic membrane was a valuable allograft tissue to promote healing and repair, clinical use of amniotic membrane diminished and failed to achieve widespread use. At the time, amniotic membrane tissue was difficult to reliably source, cleanse, preserve and handle. Additionally, fresh allografts carried a risk of infectious disease transmission such as human immunodeficiency virus (HIV) from the donor tissue. Limited processing and preservation methods also made transportation and storage of the tissue difficult [47].

However, with improvements in processing techniques and quality control of infectious disease testing, amniotic membrane tissues were reintroduced for ophthalmic applications in the 1990s. Use increased rapidly with ophthalmology becoming one of the most popular applications of the material in the late twentieth century [46]. Amniotic membrane is currently used for conjunctival reconstruction, burn treatment, pterygium repair and a number of other similar applications. Following the success of amniotic tissue in ophthalmology, adaption of preserved amniotic tissues for wound care soon followed.

3.2. Recent advances in wound care

3.2.1. Improvements in placental tissue processing

As processing techniques continued to improve, use of amniotic membrane allografts in wound care increased, as did use in dental and surgical applications. Various methods have been developed to cleanse, prepare and preserve the tissue for surgical use. Additionally, improved controls are now in place to appropriately preserve the tissue and reduce the risk of infectious disease transmission.

In the United States, human placentas are donated under informed consent, in compliance with the Food and Drug Administration's (FDA) Good Tissue Practices (GTP) and the American Association of Tissue Banks' (AATB) standards. Mothers can choose to donate their placentas following full-term, live births that result in both a healthy mother and child. Placentas are typically donated following scheduled Caesarean sections, which allow the tissue to be maintained in the aseptic field without passing through the birth canal. All donors are tested and confirmed free of infectious diseases, including HIV, human T-lymphotropic virus (HTLV), hepatitis B and C and syphilis, in accordance with the AATB standards.

Allograft tissues may be processed using a variety of techniques. For example, many allografts (harvested from another human tissue donor) and xenografts (harvested from animal tissues) are fully decellularized in order to remove immunogenic cellular components and prevent immune rejection by the recipient. The process of decellularization intentionally washes out immunoreactive cellular components including bioactive regulatory factors, leaving a structurally intact but biologically inert extracellular matrix scaffold. While decellularization is necessary to prevent host rejection in xenograft tissues (such as porcine small intestinal submucosa or urinary bladder) and nonimmunologically privileged human allograft tissues (such as human dermis), fetal-derived placental tissue allografts are immunologically privileged tissues. Fetal placental tissues contain low levels of HLA antigens and do not elicit immune rejection. Therefore, placental tissues may be gently cleansed to remove blood and hazardous materials, while preserving the natural biological activity of the tissue for transplantation without complete decellularization.

Human amniotic membranes have increased in popularity as barrier membranes to promote healing of dermal, ophthalmic and surgical wounds, partly due to their immunologically privileged properties [47]. To provide a product for patient use, allograft tissues require preservation techniques to allow for transportation, storage and off-the-shelf usage. The most common method to preserve tissue grafts and prevent degradation is through cryopreservation or freezing. Freezing tissue can prevent degradation by reducing enzymatic and chemical activity in the tissues and inhibiting the growth of microorganisms. However, cryopreserved grafts are often cumbersome to transport and store, requiring temperature-controlled conditions such as liquid nitrogen, dry ice, or large freezers, often at -80°C or below. Cryopreserved grafts also are commonly stored in cryoprotectants, such as dimethylsulfoxide (DMSO) and glycerol, added to mitigate the effects of ice crystal formation within the tissues, which can destroy cellular membranes and disrupt tissue matrix. These cryoprotectants, however, can be cytotoxic at high concentrations or extended exposure times and must be thoroughly rinsed from the tissues prior to application on patients.

An increasingly popular alternative to cryopreservation is tissue dehydration. Tissue can be dehydrated under heat, open air, or freeze drying (lyophilization). By removing residual moisture, tissue can be preserved by reducing activity of soluble chemical reactions and water-dependent enzymatic activity and inhibiting the viability of microorganisms in a low moisture environment. Dehydration preserves tissue without the need for freezers, dry ice, or liquid nitrogen and certain methods of dehydration have been shown to retain equivalent or superior biological activity compared to cryopreservation, with the benefits of being shipped and stored at ambient conditions. Dehydrated tissues are also typically stronger and easier to handle than wet tissues. Though dehydration may alter the tissue's microstructure by causing the matrix to become more compact in the absence of water, by preserving the native tissue matrix proteins the dehydrated tissue can be rehydrated in the wound environment to return the tissue to its original state.

Following dehydration, human amniotic membrane tissue is easy to handle and can be stored at ambient conditions with a shelf-life of up to 5 years, while preserving the structural integrity and biochemical activity of native amniotic membrane. Even though dehydration renders amniotic cells nonviable, these cells remain structurally intact, including the cellular and pericellular components that play essential roles in regulating biological activity. Retention of bioactive factors is thought to be critical to the clinical efficacy of amniotic tissue allografts in wound repair and tissue regeneration. Therefore, harsh cleansing processes that wash bioactive material out of the grafts may greatly reduce the cytokine content and diminish the clinical efficacy of the naturally derived tissues.

An additional benefit of tissue dehydration is that the allografts can be terminally sterilized to reduce the risk of infectious disease from the donor tissue. While all allograft tissues are aseptically processed to reduce the risk of bacterial or viral contamination, dehydrated tissues can be terminally sterilized using techniques such as gamma ray or electron beam irradiation to further reduce the risk of disease transmission. Though high levels of radiation may potentially crosslink or denature proteins within tissues, terminally sterilized amniotic membranes allografts have been proven to retain biological activity both clinically and through *in vitro* experiments [3, 5]. These data suggest that sterilization does not significantly diminish the bioactivity of amniotic membrane allografts and is worthwhile to ensure maximal safety to patients.

Each tissue processing technique has differing advantages and disadvantages based on the clinical goal of the resulting allograft tissue. However, with amniotic membrane tissue, the goal of tissue processing is to cleanse the tissue of hazardous materials in order to ensure a safe allograft product for the patient while preserving the natural properties and biological activity of the native amniotic membrane tissue to maximize efficacy and promote tissue healing. With its rapid growth, usage of amniotic membrane has now expanded to include many other promising applications in addition to wound care. It is emerging as a reparative membrane in orthopedics, neurosurgery, periodontology, gynecological surgery, general and reconstructive surgery and a number of other medical fields [47].

3.2.2. *Amniotic membrane allograft composition*

Due to remarkable clinical success, use of placental tissue allografts has largely focused on amniotic membrane to date. Amniotic membrane allografts can comprise single-layer amnion tissue, or the amnion can be combined with the chorion layer to form a laminated graft. Beginning with success in ophthalmological applications in which a thin, unobtrusive membrane is often desired, single-layer amnion grafts have increased in popularity to promote healing of dermal wounds. More recently, laminated membranes of amnion and chorion have also been developed to provide thicker, more substantial grafts. In particular, MiMedx Group, Inc. (Marietta, GA) uses a proprietary, patent-protected PURION® Process to manufacture dehydrated human amnion/chorion membrane (dHACM) allografts (EpiFix®). Hematoxylin and eosin (H&E) staining of dHACM, which stains cell nuclei dark blue and stains connective tissue and cytoplasm pink, is shown in **Figure 2**. Because the chorion is dissected from the amniotic sac and not from the placental disc or from the chorionic plate to produce these dHACM grafts, the chorion tissue in PURION® Processed dHACM is nonmaternally derived and is immunologically privileged with a low risk of eliciting an immune response.

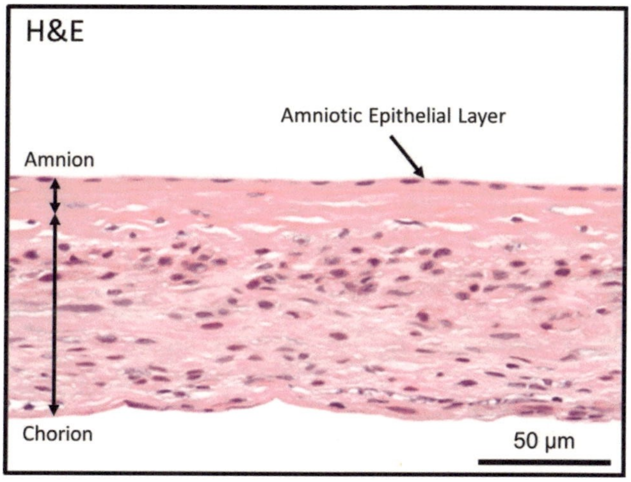

Figure 2. Hematoxylin and eosin (H&E) staining of dehydrated human amnion/chorion membrane (dHACM).

A significant advantage of including chorion tissue in an amniotic membrane allograft is that the chorion is approximately three to four times thicker than the amnion layer alone while containing a similar distribution of bioactive growth factors [48]. Therefore, lamination of the amnion and chorion layers results in a thicker graft with easier handling characteristics and significantly greater total content of growth factors and cytokines than single layer, amnion-only grafts. By preserving the content of amniotic membrane tissue and utilizing the thicker chorion layer, PURION® Processed dHACM grafts have been shown to contain as much as 20-fold greater levels of growth factors and cytokines than other amnion-only allografts [48].

Various amniotic membrane allografts have also been micronized into particulate forms or suspended in fluid to allow injection of the grafts for sports medicine and wound applications.

These injectable tissues have been used in capsular joints to relieve pain and promote soft tissue healing, as well as to modulate inflammation and promote healing of microtears, such as in plantar fasciitis [49].

3.2.3. Regulation of placental tissue allografts

In the United States, placental tissues, including amniotic membrane allografts, are commonly regulated by the FDA as human cells, tissues and cellular and tissue-based products (HCT/Ps) under Section 361 of the Public Health Service (PHS) Act. Tissues regulated as Section 361 HCT/Ps do not require FDA clearance or approval; however, the HCT/P allografts are required to be in compliance with the FDA's current Good Tissue Practices (cGTP) regulations and 21 Code of Federal Regulations (CFR) Part 1270 and 21 CFR Part 1271. These standards are important to prevent introduction, transmission, or spread of communicable diseases. Regulations require that manufactured products are registered with the FDA and that stringent donor eligibility requirements are in place for donor screening and testing of relevant communicable diseases. cGTP establishes guidelines for manufacturing methods, facilities and controls to ensure that HCT/Ps do not contain communicable disease agents, are not contaminated and do not become contaminated during processing. Tissue processing sites must also be registered as tissue banks with the AATB.

Tissues regulated as Section 361 HCT/Ps are required to be "minimally manipulated" human tissues, meaning that processing cannot alter the original relevant characteristics of the tissue and that the tissue cannot be combined with another article. These HCT/P tissues are intended for homologous use, meaning that they perform the same basic functions in the recipient as the donor and they do not have a systemic effect. The 361 HCT/P regulatory pathway allows naturally derived tissues to be transplanted for use, as long as they are safe and used in an appropriate manner. In accordance with these regulations, amniotic membrane allografts act as barriers to modulate inflammation, reduce scar tissue formation and enhance healing.

3.3. Recent clinical data in wound care

To date, clinical data on placental tissues has focused largely on amniotic membrane allografts. Amniotic membrane has proven to be an effective therapy to promote epithelialization, modulate inflammation, inhibit protease activity and enhance wound healing [19, 46]. Another promising characteristic of placental tissue is the ability to reduce fibrous scar tissue formation, as fetal tissue and the fetal environment are known to support scarless healing, though the molecular mechanisms are not yet fully understood [50].

Though many case studies exist documenting the use of amniotic membrane allografts in wound care, the number of prospective, randomized controlled clinical trials (RCTs) on placental tissues are currently limited. However, several RCTs have demonstrated the efficacy of amniotic membrane allografts in healing of chronic wounds. In particular, PURION® Processed dehydrated human amnion/chorion membrane (dHACM) allografts (EpiFix®, MiMedx Group, Inc.) have demonstrated promising clinical results in a number of randomized clinical trials, including studies in diabetic foot ulcers (DFUs) and venous leg ulcers

http://dx.doi.org/10.5772/65321

(VLU) [3, 4]. A number of additional studies from various sponsors are registered on ClinicalTrials.gov and are currently ongoing [51].

3.3.1. *Amnion/chorion allografts in healing of diabetic foot ulcers*

A prospective RCT examined healing rates of diabetic foot ulcers (DFUs) treated with a biweekly application of PURION® Processed dHACM allografts (EpiFix®, MiMedx Group, Inc.; $n = 13$), compared to DFUs treated with a standard of care regimen of moist wound therapy alone ($n = 12$). Results demonstrated a statistically significant improvement in healing with 77% and 92% of wounds treated with dHACM completely healed at 4 and 6 weeks, respectively, compared to only 0% and 8% of wounds healed in standard of care controls [3]. Wounds were also reduced in size by an average of 97.1 ± 7.0% and 98.4 ± 5.8% after 4 and 6 weeks, respectively, with dHACM treatment, compared to 32.0 ± 47.3% and -1.8 ± 0.3% reduction in standard of care patients. Despite the relatively small number of patients included in this study, statistically significant differences were observed between treatment groups due to the drastic effect of dHACM on healing rates and the trial was terminated early at 25 patients since the investigator felt that further treatment of patients with standard of care alone would be potentially unethical.

To further support these promising results, patients that failed to heal with standard of care treatment were subsequently treated with a biweekly application of dHACM allografts ($n = 11$). In this crossover study of patients, 55% patients demonstrated complete healing by 4 weeks, along with 64% by 6 weeks and 91% by 12 weeks with application of PURION® Processed dHACM [52]. Additionally, wounds that healed after dHACM treatment in the original and crossover populations were examined for long-term durability, 9–12 months after primary healing. Of the patients that healed in response to dHACM and returned for follow-up ($n = 18$), 94.4% remained fully healed without wound recurrence at the same location [53]. These results reinforce that a significant healing response was observed in chronic DFUs in response to dHACM treatment.

In a separate study to determine the optimal dosing frequency for application of PURION® Processed dHACM allografts, a weekly application ($n = 20$) was compared with biweekly applications ($n = 20$) of dHACM (EpiFix®, MiMedx Group, Inc.) in a prospective, randomized clinical study. The weekly application of dHACM healed diabetic foot ulcers in a mean time to complete healing of 2.4 ± 1.8 weeks, compared to 4.1 ± 2.9 weeks with biweekly applications [54]. Complete healing occurred in 90% of wounds by 4 weeks in the weekly group, while 50% of wounds completely healed by 4 weeks with biweekly treatment. Therefore, these results indicate that with weekly applications wounds healed in approximately half of the time and using a similar number of grafts applied as the biweekly application, even though overall 92.5% of ulcers completely healed during the 12-week study period with dHACM treatment. These results further demonstrated that dHACM allografts are an effective treatment to promote healing in diabetic foot ulcers and suggest that wounds treated with a weekly application of dHACM heal more rapidly than with biweekly application.

3.3.2. Single-layer amnion allografts in healing of diabetic foot ulcers

Only two other amniotic membrane products of note have been used in published prospective RCTs in wounds to date. Using a human viable wound matrix (hVWM; Grafix®, Osiris Therapeutics, Inc., Columbia, MD) composed of cryopreserved amnion, DFUs were treated weekly with hVWM ($n = 50$), compared to standard of care treatment ($n = 47$), in a prospective, randomized multicenter trial. In this study, 62.0% of patients treated with hVWM experienced complete wound closure after 12 weeks, compared to 21.3% of standard of care patients [55]. Among the study participants that healed, ulcers remained closed in 82.1% of patients in the hVWM group and 70% in the control group after an additional 12 weeks.

Dehydrated amniotic membrane allograft (DAMA; AMNIOEXCEL®, Derma Sciences, Inc., Princeton, NJ) composed of dehydrated amnion was also examined in a prospective, randomized multicenter trial for treatment of DFUs. DFUs were treated weekly with DAMA ($n = 15$), compared to standard of care ($n = 14$). In this study, 33% of the subjects treated with DAMA achieved complete wound closure after 6 weeks, compared with 0% of the patients in the standard of care cohort [56].

These studies using single-layer amnion allografts did not achieve healing rates as high or speed of healing as rapid as laminated PURION® Processed amnion/chorion grafts; however, it is difficult to compare healing rates across multiple studies due to the differing patient populations and treatment regimens involved. To compare the effectiveness of therapies, a comparative effectiveness trial is required to compare allograft efficacy in a controlled manner. Nevertheless, the results of these clinical trials indicate that amniotic membrane grafts are safe to use and accelerate healing of chronic DFUs.

3.3.3. Comparative effectiveness of amnion/chorion allografts with bioengineered skin substitute in diabetic ulcers

In a prospective, randomized multicenter comparative effectiveness study, weekly applications of PURION® Processed dHACM (EpiFix®, MiMedx Group, Inc.; $n = 20$) was compared with bioengineered skin substitute (Apligraf®, Organogenesis, Inc., Canton, MA; $n = 20$) and standard of care (collagen-alginate dressing; $n = 20$) for treatment of chronic lower extremity diabetic ulcers. After 4 and 6 weeks, 85 and 95% of ulcers treated with dHACM, respectively, achieved complete wound closure, which was significantly higher than for patients receiving the bioengineered skin substitute which healed 35 and 45% of wounds, respectively, or standard of care treatment with 30 and 35%, respectively [57]. Median time to healing with dHACM was 13 days, compared to 49 days with bioengineered skin substitute and the mean number of dHACM grafts used was 2.5 applications at an average cost of $1669 per patient, compared to 6.2 bioengineered skin substitute grafts used at a cost of $9216, indicating that costs were significantly less for dHACM than the bioengineered skin substitute by a factor of five. These results reaffirm both the efficacy and cost effectiveness of dHACM amniotic membrane allografts to promote healing in chronic diabetic ulcers in comparison with a leading skin substitute.

3.3.4. Amnion/chorion allografts in healing of venous leg ulcers

To examine the effectiveness of amniotic membrane allografts in difficult to heal venous leg ulcers (VLUs), a prospective, randomized multicenter trial evaluated the safety and efficacy of PURION® Processed dHACM (EpiFix®, MiMedx Group, Inc.) in the treatment of VLUs. Patients with VLUs were treated with either one or two applications of dHACM (n = 53) with multilayer compression therapy (MLCT) versus a standard of care (n = 31) of MLCT alone and patients were examined for an outcome of ≥40% reduction of wound size at 4 weeks, which is a surrogate endpoint found throughout the literature as a strong indicator of healing. After 4 weeks, 62% of patients receiving dHACM and 32% of those receiving MLCT alone demonstrated ≥40% wound closure [4]. Wounds treated with dHACM allograft were reduced in size by a mean of 48.1% after 4 weeks, compared to 19.0% for standard of care controls. This 40% wound closure endpoint was later validated with data demonstrating that 80% of all patients demonstrating ≥40% closure of VLUs after 4 weeks progressed to complete closure within 24 weeks, compared to only 33% of patients who demonstrated <40% healing after 4 weeks [58]. Additionally, 79.5% of patients treated with dHACM reported a reduction in pain using a visual analogue scale (VAS), compared to 52.4% of patients receiving MLCT alone. The results of this trial showed that VLUs treated with only one or two applications of dHACM experienced an accelerated rate of healing which encouraged long-term wound closure and that dHACM allografts significantly improve healing of venous leg ulcers. Together with the DFU data presented above, these clinical trials clearly demonstrate that amniotic membrane allografts promote a more rapid rate of healing in treatment of a variety of dermal wounds.

4. Scientific mechanisms to promote healing using placental tissues

Placental tissue allografts have rapidly escalated as promising advanced wound care therapies; therefore, several scientific studies have sought to improve understanding of the molecular mechanisms by which placental tissue grafts improve healing. While the cellular and molecular mechanisms by which placental tissue allografts enhance healing are still under investigation, scientific and clinical research suggest that placental tissues, including amniotic membrane, umbilical cord and amniotic fluid, possess significant promise as advanced therapies to promote healing of wounds through bioactive modulation of cellular responses and wound environments.

In particular, research has focused on the ability of amniotic membrane tissues as immunologically privileged barriers to modulate inflammation, reduce scarring and enhance healing. PURION® Processed dehydrated human amnion/chorion amniotic membrane (dHACM) allografts (EpiFix®, MiMedx Group, Inc.) have been shown to promote proliferation, migration and modulate cytokine secretion by a variety of cells involved in wound healing.

4.1. Growth factor content

To date, over 226 growth factors, cytokines, chemokines and regulatory proteins have been identified in PURION® Processed dHACM allografts, as shown in **Figure 3** [21]. These

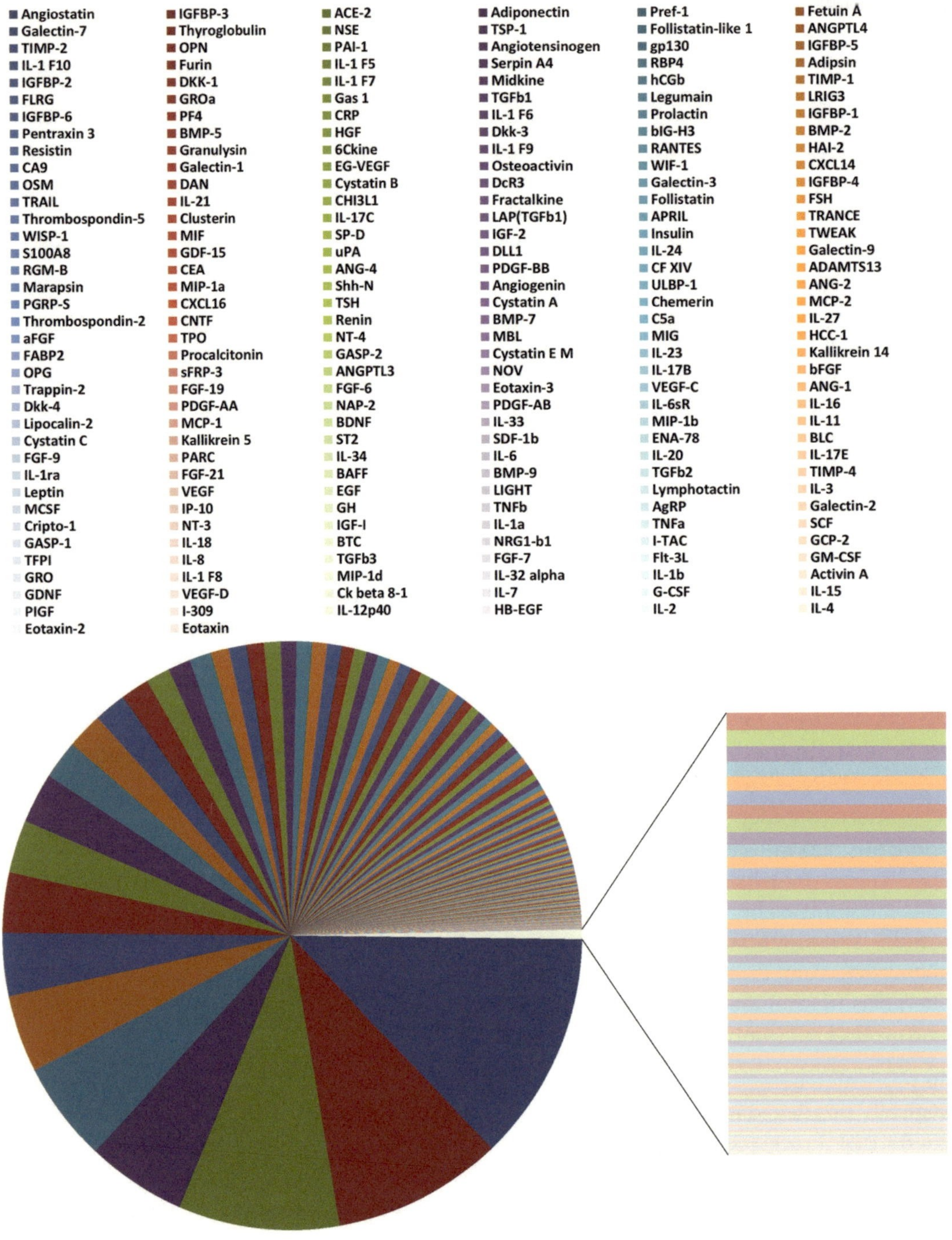

Figure 3. Relative content of 226 various growth factors, cytokines and regulatory molecules identified in dehydrated human amnion/chorion membrane (dHACM) allografts. Factors are listed in order of decreasing abundance, reading from left to right.

molecules, which include a wide array of growth factors, immunomodulatory cytokines and chemokines and TIMPs, possess important roles in regulating fetal development and pregnancy and therefore may modulate various stages of tissue healing and regeneration. dHACM allografts deliver these bioactive molecules into the wound environment, as an initial fraction of these critical factors are freely soluble and elute out from the grafts, while the remaining fraction remains bound within the tissue extracellular matrix [5]. As the remaining tissue is resorbed over time by matrix metalloproteinases in the wound, the growth factors bound to the extracellular matrix can be released into the surrounding tissue, providing a sustained release of growth factors during the tissue regeneration process.

These results suggest that dHACM grafts deliver active growth factors, cytokines, chemokines and regulatory proteins including an abundance of protease inhibitors that are essential for soft tissue healing [72]. In particular, modulation of inflammation is critical during the early stages of wound repair and dHACM contains an array of immunomodulatory cytokines and chemokines that regulate the activity of immune cells, suggesting dHACM allografts deliver a balance of inflammatory regulators which may modulate the inflammation response within healing wounds.

4.2. Cell proliferation

PURION® Processed dHACM has also been shown to promote cellular proliferation of a variety of cell types involved in wound healing, including human dermal fibroblasts, microvascular endothelial cells and adult stem cells such as bone marrow mesenchymal stem cells (BM-MSCs), adipose-derived stem cells (ADSCs) and hematopoietic stem cells (HSCs) *in vitro*. When cultured in the presence of soluble extracts of dHACM tissue containing a cocktail of naturally derived growth factors and cytokines from amniotic tissue, dHACM was shown to stimulate proliferation *in vitro* in all of these cells types relevant to healing and repair [5–7]. These results demonstrate that dHACM directly causes human dermal fibroblasts, microvascular endothelial cells, mesenchymal stem cells, adipose-derived stem cells and hematopoietic stem cells to proliferate *in vitro* by releasing growth factors that activate the proliferative response and therefore may act by amplifying the respective populations of these cells in wound environments.

4.3. Stem cell migration

In addition to promoting cell proliferation, PURION® Processed dHACM was shown to recruit migration of adult stem cells, including mesenchymal stem cells, adipose-derived stem cells and hematopoietic stem cells *in vitro* and *in vivo*. Using *in vitro* assays, dHACM promoted chemotactic migration of MSCs across porous membranes toward dHACM tissue and accelerated migration of MSCs and ADSCs in closure of cell-free zones [5, 7]. The ability to promote chemotactic stem cell migration was confirmed *in vivo* using a murine ischemic wound model. Increased numbers of MSCs and HSCs were measured at the site of subcutaneous dHACM implantation using flow cytometry, compared to sham wounds without dHACM [5, 8]. Additionally, a parabiosis model was used in which the circulation of a green fluorescent protein (GFP^+) mouse was linked with a wild-type mouse as shown in **Figure 4**.

Flow cytometry and immunohistochemistry identified GFP$^+$ stem cells at sites of neovascularization within implanted dHACM grafts in wild-type mice (**Figure 4**, blue), compared to sham and acellular dermal matrix (ADM) controls, indicating that stem cells were recruited through the blood circulation toward the dHACM grafts [8]. Cellular expression of stromal derived factor 1α (SDF-1α), a known stem cell recruiting factor, was also upregulated after dHACM implantation, which may attract additional cells to the site and further promote repair. Stem cells are pivotal cells that are normally recruited to sites of injury, where they mount a multifaceted cascade regulating inflammatory mechanisms, angiogenesis and tissue regeneration. Therefore, these data indicate that dHACM may stimulate healing by recruiting the patient's own reservoir of reparative stem cells from the circulation toward sites of implantation within healing wounds, thereby acting as a "stem cell magnet" to amplify stem cell populations within healing wounds.

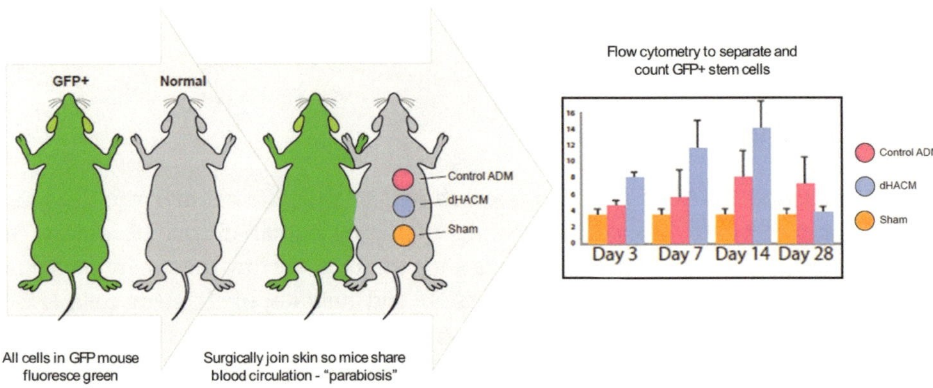

Figure 4. Parabiosis of a GFP$^+$ mouse with a normal mouse demonstrated the ability of dehydrated human amnion/chorion membrane (dHACM) to recruit circulating stem cells from the bloodstream. Greater numbers of GFP$^+$ stem cells were identified in sites of subcutaneous dHACM implantation (blue) by flow cytometry, compared to sham (orange) and acellular dermal matrix (ADM; pink) controls.

4.4. Secretion of immunomodulatory, angiogenic and tissue promoting cytokines

PURION® Processed dHACM has also been shown to modulate cellular activity by stimulating the secretion of cytokines by fibroblasts, vascular endothelial cells and adult stem cells, including secretion of immunomodulatory, angiogenic and tissue growth promoting cytokines [6, 7, 59]. In particular, the role of stem cells in healing has recently focused on the paracrine signaling properties of these cells, including their influence on the inflammatory status of injured tissues. ADSCs, BM-MSCs and HSCs were shown to modulate secretion of a number of cytokines involved in immunoregulation and mitogenesis in response to dHACM extracts, including chemokines and proteins related to leukocyte migration, immunomodulatory cytokines and mitogenic growth factors and proteins related to tissue growth [7]. These results indicate that in addition to the growth factors and cytokines released from dHACM tissue into the wound, dHACM continues to amplify these paracrine signals by inducing resident cells to produce additional regenerative growth factors and this balance of regulatory cues may modulate the wound environment to promote healing.

Although stem cells in diabetic patients are believed to be impaired and less responsive due to hyperglycemia and reduced cytokine bioavailability resulting from the disease state, PURION® Processed dHACM was capable of stimulating ADSCs from type I and type II diabetic donors to proliferate, migrate and modulate gene expression and secretion of immunomodulatory cytokines *in vitro*, similar to levels observed by ADSCs from a healthy donor [60]. These results demonstrate that while stem cells from diabetic donors may have decreased capacities for healing, contributing to the development of chronic wounds, stem cells derived from diabetic patients were capable of responding to treatment with dHACM, suggesting that dHACM treatment may stimulate stem cell activity to promote healing in diabetic ulcers.

4.5. Angiogenesis

An array of angiogenic cytokines have been identified in PURION® Processed dHACM and dHACM was shown to stimulate human dermal microvascular endothelial cells *in vitro*. dHACM caused endothelial cells to proliferate, migrate and induce production of over 30 angiogenic factors *in vitro* [6]. Additionally, following subcutaneous implantation in a murine ischemic wound model, a steady increase in microvessels in dHACM implants was observed *in vivo* over a 4-week period. These levels were equivalent to healthy and healed skin indicating a dynamic intra-dHACM implant neovascular process. Angiogenesis is paramount during the late inflammatory and proliferative phases of wound healing since chronic wounds are commonly associated with poor circulation and vascularization. Therefore, these results demonstrate that dHACM grafts: (1) contain angiogenic growth factors retaining biological activity; (2) promote amplification of angiogenic cues by inducing endothelial cell proliferation and migration and by upregulating production of endogenous angiogenic growth factors by endothelial cells; and (3) support the formation of blood vessels *in vivo*.

Together, these *in vitro* and *in vivo* scientific results strongly suggest that PURION® Processed dHACM is intimately involved with modulation of the cellular environments in wounds to elicit an improved healing response and the reparative attributes of dHACM allografts are further supported by the numerous published clinical trials on their use to promote healing of diabetic foot ulcers and venous leg ulcers. Through the delivery of a diverse cocktail of biologically active signals into the wound environment, PURION® Processed dHACM tissues directly promote cell proliferation and migration to amplify cell populations in the wound and stimulate cytokine secretion of important growth factors and immunomodulatory regulators by these cells. Collectively these cellular cues work together to stimulate stem cell activity, angiogenesis and modulation of inflammation and may reset the wound environment from one of a stalled, chronic state to an acute wound that can progress through the normal healing stages of inflammation, proliferation and remodeling. Though these mechanisms may be characteristic of other placental tissues and amniotic membrane allografts, it should be noted that these cellular responses were demonstrated using PURION® Processed dehydrate human amnion/chorion membrane (dHACM) allografts (EpiFix®, MiMedx Group, Inc.).

4.6. Scientific data from single-layer amnion allografts

Though limited in number, to date, two single-layer amniotic membrane products have been examined for their ability to modulate cellular activity during wound healing and the results have been published in peer-reviewed scientific journals. A study using devitalized, cryopreserved amnion (TissueTech, Inc., Miami, FL) demonstrated the ability of amniotic membrane allografts to suppress macrophage viability and proliferation and to inhibit TGF-β1 signaling, supporting the immunomodulatory properties of amniotic membrane tissue [61]. Additionally, a series of studies on viable, cryopreserved amnion (Grafix®, Osiris Therapeutics, Inc.) demonstrated that amniotic membrane allografts possess angiogenic, antiinflammatory and antioxidant capacity, as indicated by *in vitro* experiments of endothelial cell migration and tube formation [62]; peripheral blood mononuclear cell (PBMC) secretion of tumor necrosis factor α (TNF-α), IL-1α and IL-10 and inhibition collagenase [63]; and reduced oxidant-induced damage in dermal fibroblasts and migration of fibroblasts and keratinocytes [64].

5. Promise of placental tissues for wound healing

Though scientific and clinical data have focused largely on amniotic membrane tissues thus far, other placental tissues are generating significant interest as tissue allografts to support healing of wounds. Due to the structural and functional differences of the placental tissues, these tissues may provide alternative treatment regimens. For example, the structural and biological composition of umbilical cord and amniotic fluid suggests that they may facilitate additional applications beyond amniotic membrane grafts including thicker grafts to better facilitate suturing or liquid grafts for delivery through injection.

Umbilical cord allografts have begun to increase usage as wound therapies (e.g., EpiCord™, MiMedx Group, Inc.). Umbilical cord is composed of Wharton's jelly with a high content of hyaluronic acid, as well as a number of regulatory growth factors and cytokines. Due to the increased thickness of the umbilical cord matrix relative to amniotic membrane, umbilical cord may be easier to handle and suture into place when a thicker graft is desired for deeper wounds, while retaining a similar array of bioactive proteins to promote healing.

As a liquid allograft, amniotic fluid can be delivered in a unique form including injection into wounds or joint spaces (e.g., OrthoFlo, MiMedx Group, Inc.). Amniotic fluid is composed of a complex solution of growth factors, cytokines, proteins, carbohydrates, lipids, hormones, electrolytes, hyaluronic acid, as well as other nutrients, which function to protect and cushion, modulate inflammation and enhance mobility *in utero* [22, 24, 65]. Though clinical data on amniotic fluid are limited, a number of cases have demonstrated that injection of amniotic fluid is safe and anecdotal results suggest that amniotic fluid reduces pain and promotes healing [66, 67]. Additional *in vivo* preclinical models have demonstrated that amniotic fluid promotes healing in a variety of applications including healing of wounds, burns, bone, cartilage, tendon and nerves [68–71].

The placental disc is a rich source of fetal nutrients; however, because it contains both maternal and fetal components, the placental disc tissue requires decellularization to prevent immuno-

http://dx.doi.org/10.5772/65321

logical rejection following implantation and wound healing applications are generally limited to the use of the decellularized placental disc matrix. Decellularization removes biologically active components; however, with appropriate processing methods, the extracellular matrix can be preserved. The placental disc is a rich source of collagen, particularly collagen type I; therefore, placental collagen is currently under investigation to develop collagen-based scaffolds in the form of sponges or void fillers (e.g., AmnioFill™, MiMedx Group, Inc.). Additionally in an unrelated application, purified placental collagen has also been used to manufacture cross-linked collagen fibers for use as sutures and tendon repair devices (e.g., CollaFix™, MiMedx Group, Inc.).

Overall, the fetal environment has tremendous capacity to support and guide tissue development and enable scarless healing and placental tissue including the umbilical cord, amniotic fluid and amniotic membrane actively regulate and maintain the composition and structure of the fetal environment. These tissues are also immunologically privileged as barrier tissues that separate the mother from the fetus and support immunological tolerance. These complex, nutrient-rich tissues are created biologically to support growth during pregnancy and clinical results indicate that they possess significant promise to enhance wound healing by delivering cytokines, which alter the wound environment and stimulate endogenous cells to reset the natural wound healing process.

The unique characteristics of placental tissue allografts make them promising therapies for wound care and soft tissue healing, including for a variety of chronic and acute wounds, burns, plastic and reconstructive surgery, as well as various surgical and sports medicine applications. Placental tissue allografts provide a bioactive therapy for treatment of complex wounds where standard of care treatment is not sufficient, with the ability to modulate inflammation and reduce scar tissue formation. Placental tissue also has specific advantages over many other available bioactive therapies, including reduced cost, an abundance of donor tissue, ease of handling and being immunologically privileged. While the exact mechanisms by which placental tissue allografts promote healing remain under investigation, *in vitro* and *in vivo* research suggests that they alter cellular activity within the wound environment by modulating inflammation, promoting cellular migration and proliferation and stimulating stem cell activity. These cellular responses may then reset the healing trajectory and encourage progression through the natural stages of inflammation, proliferation and remodeling to enhance wound healing.

Author details

Jeremy J. Lim* and Thomas J. Koob

*Address all correspondence to: jlim@mimedx.com

MiMedx Group, Inc., Marietta, GA, USA

References

[1] Gude NM, Roberts CT, Kalionis B, King RG. Growth and function of the normal human placenta. Thrombosis Research. 2004;114(5–6):397–407.

[2] Warning JC, McCracken SA, Morris JM. A balancing act: mechanisms by which the fetus avoids rejection by the maternal immune system. Reproduction. 2011;141(6):715–24.

[3] Zelen CM, Serena TE, Denoziere G, Fetterolf DE. A prospective randomised comparative parallel study of amniotic membrane wound graft in the management of diabetic foot ulcers. International Wound Journal. 2013;10(5):502–507.

[4] Serena TE, Carter MJ, Le LT, Sabo MJ, DiMarco DT, EpiFix VLUSG. A multicenter, randomized, controlled clinical trial evaluating the use of dehydrated human amnion/chorion membrane allografts and multilayer compression therapy vs. multilayer compression therapy alone in the treatment of venous leg ulcers. Wound Repair and Regeneration: Official Publication of the Wound Healing Society [and] the European Tissue Repair Society. 2014;22(6):688–693.

[5] Koob TJ, Rennert R, Zabek N, Massee M, Lim JJ, Temenoff JS, et al. Biological properties of dehydrated human amnion/chorion composite graft: implications for chronic wound healing. International Wound Journal. 2013;10(5):493–500.

[6] Koob TJ, Lim JJ, Massee M, Zabek N, Rennert R, Gurtner G, et al. Angiogenic properties of dehydrated human amnion/chorion allografts: therapeutic potential for soft tissue repair and regeneration. Vascular Cell. 2014;6:10.

[7] Massee M, Chinn K, Lei J, Lim JJ, Young CS, Koob TJ. Dehydrated human amnion/chorion membrane regulates stem cell activity in vitro. Journal of Biomedical Materials Research Part B, Applied Biomaterials. 2016;104(7):1495–1503.

[8] Maan ZN, Rennert RC, Koob TJ, Januszyk M, Li WW, Gurtner GC. Cell recruitment by amnion chorion grafts promotes neovascularization. Journal of Surgical Research. 2015;193(2):953–962.

[9] Vinketova K, Mourdjeva M, Oreshkova T. Human decidual stromal cells as a component of the implantation niche and a modulator of maternal immunity. Journal of Pregnancy. 2016;2016:8689436.

[10] Benirschke K, Burton GJ, Baergen RN. Pathology of the Human Placenta. 6th ed. New York: Springer-Verlag Berlin Heidelberg; 2012. 941 p.

[11] Chen CP, Aplin JD. Placental extracellular matrix: gene expression, deposition by placental fibroblasts and the effect of oxygen. Placenta. 2003;24(4):316–325.

[12] Wang Y, Zhao S. Cell Types of the Placenta. Vascular Biology of the Placenta. Integrated Systems Physiology: From Molecules to Function to Disease. San Rafael, CA: Morgan & Claypool Life Sciences; 2010.

[13] Bankowski E, Sobolewski K, Romanowicz L, Chyczewski L, Jaworski S. Collagen and glycosaminoglycans of Wharton's jelly and their alterations in EPH-gestosis. European Journal of Obstetrics, Gynecology and Reproductive Biology. 1996;66(2):109–117.

[14] Franc S, Rousseau JC, Garrone R, van der Rest M, Moradi-Ameli M. Microfibrillar composition of umbilical cord matrix: characterization of fibrillin, collagen VI and intact collagen V. Placenta. 1998;19(1):95–104.

[15] Wang HS, Hung SC, Peng ST, Huang CC, Wei HM, Guo YJ, et al. Mesenchymal stem cells in the Wharton's jelly of the human umbilical cord. Stem Cells. 2004;22(7):1330–1337.

[16] Sobolewski K, Malkowski A, Bankowski E, Jaworski S. Wharton's jelly as a reservoir of peptide growth factors. Placenta. 2005;26(10):747–752.

[17] Parry S, Strauss JF. Premature rupture of the fetal membranes. The New England Journal of Medicine. 1998;338(10):663–670.

[18] Dua HS, Gomes JA, King AJ, Maharajan VS. The amniotic membrane in ophthalmology. Survey of Ophthalmology. 2004;49(1):51–77.

[19] Niknejad H, Peirovi H, Jorjani M, Ahmadiani A, Ghanavi J, Seifalian AM. Properties of the amniotic membrane for potential use in tissue engineering. European Cells & Materials. 2008;15:88–99.

[20] Bourne G. The foetal membranes. A review of the anatomy of normal amnion and chorion and some aspects of their function. Postgraduate Medical Journal. 1962;38:193–201.

[21] Koob TJ, Young CS, Lim JJ, Chinn K, Massee M, Carter M, et al. A Primer on Amniotic Membrane Regenerative Healing. 3rd ed. Grand Rapids, MI: MiMedx/Color House Graphics; 2016.

[22] Underwood MA, Gilbert WM, Sherman MP. Amniotic fluid: not just fetal urine anymore. Journal of Perinatology. 2005;25(5):341–348.

[23] Nyman E, Huss F, Nyman T, Junker J, Kratz G. Hyaluronic acid, an important factor in the wound healing properties of amniotic fluid: in vitro studies of re-epithelialisation in human skin wounds. Journal of Plastic Surgery and Hand Surgery. 2013;47(2):89–92.

[24] Hui AY, McCarty WJ, Masuda K, Firestein GS, Sah RL. A systems biology approach to synovial joint lubrication in health, injury and disease. Wiley Interdisciplinary Reviews: Systems Biology and Medicine. 2012;4(1):15–37.

[25] Murphy SV, Atala A. Amniotic fluid stem cells. In: Cetrulo KJ, Cetrulo CL, Taghizadeh RR, editors. Perinatal Stem Cells. 2nd ed. Hoboken, NJ: Wiley-Blackwell; 2013. p. xviii, 301 p., 8 p. of plates.

[26] Antoniadou E, David AL. Placental stem cells. Best Practice and Research Clinical Obstetrics Gynaecology. 2016;31:13–29.

[27] Garcia-Castro IL, Garcia-Lopez G, Avila-Gonzalez D, Flores-Herrera H, Molina-Hernandez A, Portillo W, et al. Markers of pluripotency in human amniotic epithelial cells and their differentiation to progenitor of cortical neurons. PLoS One. 2015;10(12):e0146082.

[28] Kim EY, Lee KB, Kim MK. The potential of mesenchymal stem cells derived from amniotic membrane and amniotic fluid for neuronal regenerative therapy. BMB Reports. 2014;47(3):135–140.

[29] De Coppi P, Bartsch G, Jr., Siddiqui MM, Xu T, Santos CC, Perin L, et al. Isolation of amniotic stem cell lines with potential for therapy. Nature Biotechnology. 2007;25(1): 100–106.

[30] Carraro G, Perin L, Sedrakyan S, Giuliani S, Tiozzo C, Lee J, et al. Human amniotic fluid stem cells can integrate and differentiate into epithelial lung lineages. Stem Cells. 2008;26(11):2902–2911.

[31] Bieback K, Kluter H. Mesenchymal stromal cells from umbilical cord blood. Current Stem Cell Research and Therapy. 2007;2(4):310–323.

[32] Weiss ML, Troyer DL. Stem cells in the umbilical cord. Stem Cell Reviews. 2006;2(2): 155–162.

[33] Zhou C, Yang B, Tian Y, Jiao H, Zheng W, Wang J, et al. Immunomodulatory effect of human umbilical cord Wharton's jelly-derived mesenchymal stem cells on lymphocytes. Cell Immunology. 2011;272(1):33–38.

[34] Cheng T, Yang B, Li D, Ma S, Tian Y, Qu R, et al. Wharton's jelly transplantation improves neurologic function in a rat model of traumatic brain injury. Cellular and Molecular Neurobiology. 2015;35(5):641–649.

[35] Nevala-Plagemann C, Lee C, Tolar J. Placenta-based therapies for the treatment of epidermolysis bullosa. Cytotherapy. 2015;17(6):786–795.

[36] Wu KH, Mo XM, Han ZC, Zhou B. Stem cell engraftment and survival in the ischemic heart. The Annals of Thoracic Surgery. 2011;92(5):1917–1925.

[37] Hocking AM, Gibran NS. Mesenchymal stem cells: paracrine signaling and differentiation during cutaneous wound repair. Experimental Cell Research. 2010;316(14):2213–2219.

[38] Volarevic V, Arsenijevic N, Lukic ML, Stojkovic M. Concise review: mesenchymal stem cell treatment of the complications of diabetes mellitus. Stem Cells. 2011;29(1):5–10.

[39] Moll G, Alm JJ, Davies LC, von Bahr L, Heldring N, Stenbeck-Funke L, et al. Do cryopreserved mesenchymal stromal cells display impaired immunomodulatory and therapeutic properties? Stem Cells. 2014;32(9):2430–2442.

[40] Marin JJ, Macias RI, Serrano MA. The hepatobiliary-like excretory function of the placenta. A review. Placenta. 2003;24(5):431–438.

[41] King AE, Paltoo A, Kelly RW, Sallenave JM, Bocking AD, Challis JR. Expression of natural antimicrobials by human placenta and fetal membranes. Placenta. 2007;28(2-3): 161–169.

[42] Tilburgs T, Evans JH, Crespo AC, Strominger JL. The HLA-G cycle provides for both NK tolerance and immunity at the maternal-fetal interface. Proceedings of the National Academy of Sciences of the United States of America. 2015;112(43): 13312–13317.

[43] Schjenken JE, Tolosa JM, Paul JW, Clifton VL, Smith R. Mechanisms of maternal immune tolerance during pregnancy. In: Zheng J, editor. Recent Advances in Research on the Human Placenta. Rijeka, Croatia: InTech; 2012. pp. 211–242.

[44] John T. Human amniotic membrane transplantation: past, present and future. Ophthalmology Clinics of North America. 2003;16(1):43–65, vi.

[45] Davis J. Skin transplantation with a review of 550 cases at The Johns Hopkins Hospital. Johns Hopkins Medical Journal. 1910;15:307–396.

[46] Dua HS, Azuara-Blanco A. Amniotic membrane transplantation. The British Journal of Ophthalmology. 1999;83(6):748–752.

[47] Fetterolf DE, Snyder RJ. Scientific and clinical support for the use of dehydrated amniotic membrane in wound management. Wounds. 2012;24(10):299–307.

[48] Koob TJ, Lim JJ, Zabek N, Massee M. Cytokines in single layer amnion allografts compared to multilayer amnion/chorion allografts for wound healing. Journal of Biomedical Materials Research Part B, Applied Biomaterials. 2015;103(5):1133–1140.

[49] Zelen CM, Poka A andrews J. Prospective, randomized, blinded, comparative study of injectable micronized dehydrated amniotic/chorionic membrane allograft for plantar fasciitis—a feasibility study. Foot and Ankle International. 2013;34(10):1332–1339.

[50] Leavitt T, Hu MS, Marshall CD, Barnes LA, Lorenz HP, Longaker MT. Scarless wound healing: finding the right cells and signals. Cell and Tissue Research. 2016;365(3):483–493.

[51] Ilic D, Vicovac L, Nikolic M, Lazic Ilic E. Human amniotic membrane grafts in therapy of chronic non-healing wounds. British Medical Bulletin. 2016;117(1):59–67.

[52] Zelen CM. An evaluation of dehydrated human amniotic membrane allografts in patients with DFUs. Journal of Wound Care. 2013;22(7):347–348, 50–51.

[53] Zelen CM, Serena TE, Fetterolf DE. Dehydrated human amnion/chorion membrane allografts in patients with chronic diabetic foot ulcers: a long-term follow-up study. Wound Medicine. 2014;4:1–4.

[54] Zelen CM, Serena TE, Snyder RJ. A prospective, randomised comparative study of weekly versus biweekly application of dehydrated human amnion/chorion membrane allograft in the management of diabetic foot ulcers. International Wound Journal. 2014;11(2):122–128.

[55] Lavery LA, Fulmer J, Shebetka KA, Regulski M, Vayser D, Fried D, et al. The efficacy and safety of Grafix((R)) for the treatment of chronic diabetic foot ulcers: results of a multi-centre, controlled, randomised, blinded, clinical trial. International Wound Journal. 2014;11(5):554–560.

[56] Snyder RJ, Shimozaki K, Tallis A, Kerzner M, Reyzelman A, Lintzeris D, et al. A prospective, randomized, multicenter, controlled evaluation of the use of dehydrated amniotic membrane allograft compared to standard of care for the closure of chronic diabetic foot ulcer. Wounds. 2016;28(3):70–77.

[57] Zelen CM, Gould L, Serena TE, Carter MJ, Keller J, Li WW. A prospective, randomised, controlled, multi-centre comparative effectiveness study of healing using dehydrated human amnion/chorion membrane allograft, bioengineered skin substitute or standard of care for treatment of chronic lower extremity diabetic ulcers. International Wound Journal. 2015;12(6):724–732.

[58] Serena TE, Yaakov R, DiMarco D, Le L, Taffe E, Donaldson M, et al. Dehydrated human amnion/chorion membrane treatment of venous leg ulcers: correlation between 4-week and 24-week outcomes. Journal of Wound Care. 2015;24(11):530–534.

[59] Koob TJ, Lim JJ, Massee M, Zabek N, Denoziere G. Properties of dehydrated human amnion/chorion composite grafts: implications for wound repair and soft tissue regeneration. Journal of Biomedical Materials Research Part B, Applied Biomaterials. 2014;102(6):1353–1362.

[60] Massee M, Chinn K, Lim JJ, Godwin L, Young CS, Koob TJ. Type I and II diabetic adipose-derived stem cells respond in vitro to dehydrated human amnion/chorion membrane allograft treatment by increasing proliferation, migration and altering cytokine secretion. Advances in Wound Care (New Rochelle). 2016;5(2):43–54.

[61] Tan EK, Cooke M, Mandrycky C, Mahabole M, He H, O'Connell J, et al. Structural and biological comparison of cryopreserved and fresh amniotic membrane tissues. Journal of Biomaterials and Tissue Engineering. 2014;4:379–388.

[62] Duan-Arnold Y, Uveges TE, Gyurdieva A, Johnson A, Danilkovitch A. Angiogenic potential of cryopreserved amniotic membrane is enhanced through retention of all tissue components in their native state. Advances in Wound Care (New Rochelle). 2015;4(9):513–522.

[63] Duan-Arnold Y, Gyurdieva A, Johnson A, Uveges TE, Jacobstein DA, Danilkovitch A. Retention of endogenous viable cells enhances the anti-inflammatory activity of cryopreserved amnion. Advances in Wound Care (New Rochelle). 2015;4(9):523–533.

[64] Duan-Arnold Y, Gyurdieva A, Johnson A, Jacobstein DA, Danilkovitch A. Soluble factors released by endogenous viable cells enhance the antioxidant and chemoattractive activities of cryopreserved amniotic membrane. Advances in Wound Care (New Rochelle). 2015;4(6):329–338.

[65] Burns C, Hall ST, Smith R, Blackwell C. Cytokine levels in late pregnancy: Are female infants better protected against inflammation? Frontiers in Immunology. 2015;6:318.

[66] Shimberg M. The use of amniotic-fluid concentrate in orthopaedic conditions. Journal of Bone and Joint Surgery: American Volume. 1938;20(1):167–177.

[67] Bhattacharya N. Clinical use of amniotic fluid in osteoarthritis: a source of cell therapy. In: Bhattacharya N, Stubblefield P, editors. Regenerative Medicine Using Pregnancy-Specific Biological Substances. London: Springer; 2011. pp. 395–403.

[68] Bazrafshan A, Owji M, Yazdani M, Varedi M. Activation of mitosis and angiogenesis in diabetes-impaired wound healing by processed human amniotic fluid. Journal of Surgical Research. 2014;188(2):545–552.

[69] Karacal N, Kosucu P, Cobanglu U, Kutlu N. Effect of human amniotic fluid on bone healing. Journal of Surgical Research. 2005;129(2):283–287.

[70] Ozgenel GY, Filiz G, Ozcan M. Effects of human amniotic fluid on cartilage regeneration from free perichondrial grafts in rabbits. British Journal of Plastic Surgery. 2004;57(5):423–428.

[71] Ozgenel GY, Samli B, Ozcan M. Effects of human amniotic fluid on peritendinous adhesion formation and tendon healing after flexor tendon surgery in rabbits. Journal of Hand Surgery: American Volume. 2001;26(2):332–339.

[72] Lei J, Priddy LB, Lim JJ, Massee M, Koob TJ. Identification of extracellular matrix components and biological factors in micronized dehydrated human amnion/chorion membrane. Advances in Wound Care (New Rochelle). 2016, ahead of print. DOI: 10.1089/wound.2016.0699.